VOICES *of* FLOWERS

USE THE NATURAL WISDOM OF PLANTS AND FLOWERS
FOR HEALTH AND RENEWAL

Rhonda M. PallasDowney

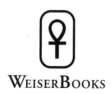

WEISERBOOKS

Medical Disclaimer

The material in this book is not intended to treat, diagnose, or prescribe. The information herein is in no way to be considered a substitute for consultation with a licensed health care practitioner.

First published in 2006 by
Red Wheel/Weiser, LLC
York Beach, ME
With offices at:
500 3rd St., #230
San Francisco, CA 94107
www.redwheelweiser.com

Library of Congress Cataloging-in-Publication Data

PallasDowney, Rhonda M.
 Voices of flowers : use the natural wisdom of plants and flowers for
health and renewal / Rhonda M. PallasDowney.
    p. cm.
Includes bibliographical references.
ISBN 1-57863-365-6 (alk. paper)
1. Flowers—Therapeutic use. 2. Symbolism of flowers. 3. Healing. I.
Title.
RX615.F55P36 2006
615'.321—dc22
                    2005027064

Typeset in Californian by Lisa Buckley Design
Photos © Rhonda PallasDowney
Photo graphic design © Susan Hook
Card design © Lisa Buckley Design

Printed in China
AP
13 12 11 10 09 08 07 06
8 7 6 5 4 3 2 1

CONTENTS

LIST OF THE FLOWERS
AND THEIR PRIMARY QUALITIES

Flower	*Quality*
1. Aster	Illumination
2. Bells-of-Ireland	Inner-Child Transformation
3. Black-Eyed Susan	Inner Peace
4. Blanketflower	Fire Dance
5. Blue Flag Iris	Stamina
6. Bouncing Bet	Mystic Union
7. Calendula	Calm
8. California Poppy	Purifier
9. Century Plant	Breakthrough
10. Chamomile	Serenity
11. Chicory	Interrelatedness
12. Cliff Rose	Positive Self-Image
13. Columbine	Divine Beauty
14. Comfrey	Service
15. Crimson Monkeyflower	Personal Power
16. Desert Larkspur	Graceful Passage
17. Desert Marigold	Flexibility
18. Desert Willow	The Empress/Compassion
19. Echinacea	Rejuvenation
20. Evening Primrose (White)	Inner Strength
21. Honeysuckle	Harmony
22. Indian Paintbrush	Creativity
23. Lupine	Pathfinder
24. Mexican Hat	Release

v

Dedication

To my mother, Bernice Reichenbach
To my beautiful family,
Curt, Sarah, Jenny, Tanya, Cortney, Adam, Victoria,
Arjuna Mateo, and Heather
And to my very special extended family,
Veronica, Jeffrey, Shandor, Jonah, Zeph, and Acou

ACKNOWLEDGMENTS

This is a place to marvel where to begin. First, I honor and give thanks to the Plants and Flowers, my teachers and my friends, for their powerful presence, their voices, the insights they give, and their medicine.

So many beautiful people in my life have inspired me, touched me, loved me, and spurred my growth. I give great thanks to my mother, Bernice Reichenbach, for her love of flowers, plants, and trees and for inspiring me unknowingly throughout my childhood. I also give thanks to my sister, Linda Burkholder, her husband Dave, and my brother, Norm Reichenbach, his wife Lin, and their families, for the many ways they have given to me over the years and for the bounty of plants and flowers growing on their farms.

I am very grateful to the Appalachian folklore mountain people of Southeastern Ohio who taught me their ways with plants. And with much appreciation, I give thanks to Matthew Wood, for his mentorship, inspiration, and love of the Plant Kingdom. I also extend my gratitude to Rosemary Gladstar for the power, love, protection, and support she gives to the earth and to all of plant life.

And to my beautiful plant sisters, Robbie Nelson, Veronica Vida, Julie Smelser, and Claudia Melton, I am so blessed to receive the support of their friendship, love, wisdom, and connection they give to me and to the Plant Kingdom. I especially give thanks to Veronica for sparking my thoughts and helping me on my path with this project, and for her beautiful poem, "May She Always Walk Among Us."

And again to Veronica and to Jeffrey, my soul cries out for our Friday night "euchre therapy" and the boundless subjects, interactions, laughter, tears, and loving friendship that always take place among the four of us. You two light up my life!

I give many thanks to my beloved, Curtis, for his support of my heart's work and for sharing his insights and inspirations with me while I wrote this book. I'm so very grateful for our experiences in nature together, for his growing appreciation of plants and flowers, and for being a gnome and guardian of earth's treasures.

And with much love, I give thanks to my daughter, Sarah, for her big heart and patience with me when I missed a few soccer tournaments and cooked fewer meals. I give thanks for both Sarah and Shandor, who inspire me in so many ways and who continue to nudge me to grow.

I am especially thankful for Namuu and Nebo, my four-legged friends who motivate me to take more walks and who share much happiness with me in nature. And also for Smoke Signals, for teaching me the ways of the cat and for her good taste in flower essences and catnip.

The gracefulness that I experienced while writing this book, I attribute to Becca Tokarczyk. Words can't express my heartfelt thanks for her healing hands and heart.

Susan Hook came into my life just in time for this project to take its form of manifestation. Susan dedicated countless hours in her graphic work, touching up my flower photos and preparing them for publishing. She has been a wonderful support and gift to me. I feel honored to have gained a new friend and am very grateful that she shared her talents with me and with you.

I extend my appreciation to Mairi Ross, another dear plant sister and author of *Smoke Plants of North America*, for her friendship and emotional support. Mairi's editing wisdom helped guide the structure of this book.

Many loving thoughts and thanks to Pk Ellis, author of *strata: mapping the voice*, and to MariJo Moore, author of *Tree Quotes*, their inspiring poetry calls out to me and deepens my soul.

To the people who made this project happen, I am ever so grateful. Many thanks to Jan Johnson for her enthusiasm and belief in this card deck at the onset and for arranging its publication; to Amy Edelstein, who did such a wonderful job copyediting; to Caroline Pincus, my managing editor, for her support, wisdom, and guidance. Kate Hartke, Liz Wood, Kathleen Fivel, and Lisa Buckley for her beautiful card designs and book cover.

ix

FOREWORD

Voices of Flowers is a jewel and reflects Rhonda PallasDowney's passion and connection with the plant world. What a delightful way to deepen our relationship with the plant kingdom. Rhonda has created another exquisite book—and a new flower card deck—on the healing power of flowers and takes us another step further into this sacred plant medicine.

The cards are a delightful addition. The card layouts will be of great use to those interested in furthering their relationship with sacred plant medicine. Once again, Rhonda opens up doorways of understanding that embrace ancient teachings from around the world and uniquely blends them with her own discoveries, creating a powerful tool of perception and healing.

Rhonda's work is both inspiring and inspired. She has cultivated a genuine, personal relationship with the plant world around her and in simple, elegant terms is able to transfer the wisdom and insight she has received to others. *Voices of Flowers* is a wonderful tool for embracing the teachings of the flowers. In essence, it invites us to slow down and smell the flowers, and by smelling, listening, and observing, we can learn from them how to create more health, harmony, and balance in our personal lives. *Voices of Flowers* is ready, at last, to begin its journey to people's hearts and souls, ready to begin its work on earth.

In Rhonda's words, "Prepare yourself for an extraordinary journey, a journey of calling in the innate wisdom and power of the Sacred Medicine of the plants and flowers."

All the best,
Rosemary Gladstar, author of *Rosemary Gladstar's Family Herbal* and founder of United Plant Savers

PREFACE

This book has been waiting to come out of the closet for nearly five years. The flowers kept talking to me about what I was going to do with them as they didn't care to be placed in their pink folder, unseen, unused, and gathering dust mites.

So I began taking the flower cards to my classes, and we would spread them out and get to know the flowers and ourselves better. Everyone loved them and wanted to know when they could have their own flower card deck. I would say something like, "That sounds like a great idea. Someday it will happen." The flowers, of course, were happy to be seen, and they loved the adoration people gave them. They liked their voices being heard, maybe because they like to give advice, or maybe just because they love seeing people become inspired.

One morning, after a restless night's sleep listening to all these plant voices talking to me and egging me on, I decided it was time to get the flower cards published. I called Georgia Hughes at New World Library, my publisher for *The Complete Book of Flower Essences*, and said "Georgia, I need to get this card deck published." Georgia gave me the phone number of her friend Jan Johnson at RedWheel Weiser and said, "Call Jan, I think she might be interested." So I did. I immediately felt a connection with Jan, and though it took us a number of months to get it together, as you can see, we finally did.

I give many heartfelt thanks to Georgia and Jan for their support and belief in my work, as well as to Nature's bounties. The flowers have been much happier, and I am sleeping better at night.

MAY SHE ALWAYS WALK AMONG US

Dedicated to Rhonda

BY VERONICA VIDA

In the high untamed desert
we spread our radiant blooms wildly
merely to be admired from a distance
We were waiting

Along the country roadside
A few glimpsed our banks brimming with brilliant hues
only to pass us by
We were waiting

Beside the flowing creeks
the water shimmered with our colors
and yet we were not seen
We were waiting

In the mountain meadows
a few paused
delighted by our fragrant richness
And yet we were still waiting

And then she came
She heeded our silent cry
She remembered our need to be seen and heard

We began to know her footsteps
in the desert, along the roadside, beside the flowing creeks, and in the meadows
We began to whisper of her coming
Eagerly awaiting her return

She sat with us
Looking deeply, exploring,
Tuning in and hearing our stories

She listened
As each of us revealed our healing medicine
She gave words to our voice and
Now many can hear and be restored

We bless and welcome her spirited footsteps
May she always walk among us

INTRODUCTION

Memories of my love of nature, plants, and flowers return to me from my childhood days. Both my parents came from large families, and many of my aunts and uncles were farmers or lived in the country. One of our family traditions each spring was to go morel mushroom hunting in the woods of different farms. While looking for the morels, I was called by the myriad of wildflowers that found their homes in the rich soil throughout the woods. They spoke to me as living, vibrant beings.

The flowers stirred my passion for life. Their gentle, eloquent beauty gave me hope and inspiration, and they gave me the strength to believe in myself. I found peace, love, and nurturing among the flowers. They were my beloved friends.

Perhaps it was my imagination, but even as a young child, I could hear the flowers and plants speak to me. As I grew older, I continued to notice and listen to the flowers and the plants. To this day, they stand by me, sing to me, embrace and welcome me. Their open invitation to adore their beauty and presence evokes a sense of purity, sacredness, vulnerability, and sometimes sadness or happiness.

I feel blessed for what I have learned about myself and others through the reflections of the plants and flowers. For example, the fiery red and powerful expression of Indian Paintbrush ignites a spark of creativity and passion within me. It feeds a depth within my soul that inspires me to write, paint, imagine, and believe.

The purple rays of an Aster reach out in invitation to embark upon the Aster's path of spirituality and joy of life. This flower offers me a sense of hope and illuminates my path. The yellow disk in its center reminds me of the mind's eye. It helps me to understand that the ability to see is beyond just the physical world. Beyond the physical is knowledge springing from a mystery that is guided by the Infinite limitless being.

The many layers and folds of a Peace Rose blossom are similar to the layers we experience in ourselves. The outer layers are looser, bigger, and easier to see, and the inner layers are tighter, smaller, and harder to peer between. If you tenderly push the inner layers back, you will find the center of the flower. The center is soft and vulnerable. Its core essence, containing the flower's soothing aroma, is subtle yet very present. It helps me to come to terms with what it truly is that I value within myself and opens my heart to receive love and feel peace.

Through these powerful relationships with plants and flowers as teachers and as friends, a doorway has opened in my life that has influenced me and all my relations. As I dive deeper into my own discoveries, I feel an expansion of awareness in my body, mind, and spirit. In that discovery, I experience an unfolding as my evolutionary path opens before me and more personal potential becomes available inside of me.

I believe that each of us is born with a special life purpose and meaning tailored to our own individuality and soul path. The ways that we think, feel, and behave influence our life choices and our life's journey. We are repeatedly tested and so learn skills and make conscious choices that lead us to realize our life's purpose. As we learn through the lessons of life, we develop skills that have meaning to us. We become connected to who we are and how we choose to live out our life. We learn that each of us is a gift to ourselves as well as to each other. As a result, our lives become richer, more meaningful, and vibrant.

Flowers and plants can help you find ways to connect with yourself. You may find yourself valuing or establishing a new relationship with a flower. This experience may help you uncover your true nature—your core essence—which may open a gateway to inner beauty, happiness, love, and well-being.

Open your mind and heart to what your eyes can't see. As you begin to experience the voice of a flower, it may reveal a message to you which contains power and mystery. Listen and allow it to help you on your path of healing and wholeness.

As you invite the innate wisdom of a flower or plant into your life, the spirit of the plant will guide you, using its own essence to show you how to reach the core essence of your being.

Peel off the layers and unfold the petals of your own evolutionary path. Allow the flowers and plants to help you discover or rediscover the depths of your innermost mysteries. Within that mystery, you may find a deeper connection with yourself and with the Circle of Life. Once you begin the journey, it is yours to walk to its end.

CHAPTER ONE

Healing Guidance from Flowers and Plants

OUR LONG HISTORY WITH PLANTS

Animals and human beings have lived a life of natural interdependence with the Plant Kingdom since they first cohabited on our planet. They are multi-faceted and offer us many gifts. They have served humans as a primary source of nourishment and have also been used for heat, shelter, clothes, weapons, and medicine. Plants were and still are used in ritual ceremony. Certain plants are believed to contain sacred and magical powers as well as natural medicinal properties.

In the history of plants and human beings, a relationship between people and plants has been formed. There is a way of relating with plants, of talking and being with plants, that is different than what is understood by the body of modern scientific knowledge. In this other way of relating, each plant speaks to us through what is called a signature. A signature is defined by the type of soil and climate a plant lives in, by its physical constituents and makeup, by its color, smell, and taste. You could think of a plant's signature as its unique expression of life.

This expression shows the personality of the plant. Just as people choose to live in certain climates such as the desert, plains, or mountains, plants grow in harmony with the climate in which they live. Desert plants require a certain ability to withstand the heat; mountain plants adapt and find their sustenance in the cooler climates. Plants express themselves through the shape of their roots, stems, and leaves and the shape and colors of their flowers. As you read this book, you will come to better understand these plants as whole beings, their personalities and their ways, their medicines and their gifts. As you take the time to look at them, to experience their wisdom and connect with their nature, you may soon discover new places within yourself.

EXPERIENCE ONENESS WITH PLANTS

Plants have wisdom to share. By joining in relationship with a plant, merging your spirit with the plant's spirit, the strength of the plant's core essence can be found and revered.

Experiencing oneness with a plant is a sign that you have reached a high level of intimacy with yourself that will only continue to open and deepen. This level of intimacy and personal growth creates an inner availability which will allow you to fully embrace and unite your own spirit with the nature spirit of the plant or flower. As you experience the nature spirit of the plant, you may experience energetic vibrations, openings, releases, and teachings of its wisdom. The power that you may experience as you connect with the nature spirit of the plant will help you discover a profound and multidimensional relationship with yourself.

You can learn to call upon the nature spirit of a plant. When you do, you will merge with its energy, taking on how the plant feels, grows, moves, breathes, lives, touches, responds, communicates, gives, and receives. Becoming one with a plant's essence, you hear the plant's voice—its songs, messages, and exaltation when its flower is at its peak.

Allow yourself to surrender to this great mystery of life. Prepare yourself for an extraordinary journey, a journey that calls in the innate wisdom and power of the sacred medicine of the plants and flowers. Hear their voices, sing their songs, speak their truths, and live as One with all Creation.

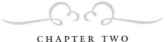

CHAPTER TWO

Flowers and Plants
and Our Chakra Energy Systems

Flowers and plants are energy systems. The energy each one emits comes from its color and essence. Each gives off distinct vibrations of sound and light. Plant spirits can speak to you through color and sound vibrations specific to each energy center within yourself. I've learned through sitting with plants over many years that the colors of the flowers, as well as the whole plant personality, have a direct correlation with the colors of the chakra energy centers of the human body. I will explain a bit about the chakras here. If you are interested in taking your study further, please refer to the section later in this book entitled, "The Seven Chakras and Their Colors: A Pathway of Wholeness", pp. 91.

The word "chakra" means "wheel of light" or "circle and movement." It refers to the subtle energy centers within the body, which actually serve as storehouses of all the various powers within our being. These energy centers relate to the gross body and its functions and are associated and connected with the parasympathetic, sympathetic, and autonomic nervous systems. The energy centers are also associated with the colors of the rainbow.

The ancient spiritual traditions of Eastern and Western mysticism, including Christianity, all recognize such an energy system. Most recognize seven major chakras or energy centers (power storehouses) within the body. For the sake of simplicity, I have focused on these seven major energy centers, although I do believe there are other energy centers within the human body and in the Light itself that is all around us. Chakras, as a universal energy system, bridge the gap between the lower and upper bodies of energy or between our lower and higher selves.

The lower three major energy centers or chakras relate to your personality self—your physical-emotional-mental makeup. This includes the way that you live, act, and function in the world. The upper three major energy centers or chakras relate to the awakening and transformation of your higher consciousness. All of the chakras interrelate and respond simultaneously with each other. Together and individually they comprise an integrated energy system. As you become more aware of yourself as a person who functions as a whole system of energy, you will experience a newfound relationship to yourself and to the world around you.

5

When I sit in silence with a plant, I resonate with the plant's wisdom and its healing properties. I notice the way it moves in the wind, its color, shape, touch, taste, and the environment in which it grows. I take on how the plant feels, grows, moves, breathes, lives, touches, responds, communicates, gives, and receives. The plant or flower has a way of relating to me that makes me feel connected to it, becoming as One with it. Through this experience, I receive guidance as to what energy center in the body the plant resonates with and how certain parts of the plant or flower resemble human nature.

Let's take the example of Indian Paintbrush. This fiery reddish-orange plant is semiparasitic, lacking a well-developed root system. Its roots grow from and depend on tissues of host plants, such as sagebrush or oak, to supply water and nutrients. Indian Paintbrush's dependence on other plants is a demonstration of its low vitality, physical weakness, and depletion of energy. The host plants that Indian Paintbrush thrives on don't appear to suffer greatly from sharing their nutrients. Yet once the Indian Paintbrush's vital force is "grounded" by burrowing its root system into the roots of the host plant, it has made a breakthrough from survival to the freedom of growing into its own creative and vibrant form.

The roots of the Indian Paintbrush burrowing into the roots of other plants, in addition to its reddish-orange fiery colors, represent both the first and second chakra energy centers. Indian Paintbrush may help you to understand and identify your own roots, where you came from genetically, and also help you understand the roots that connect you to your own spiritual heritage. From this vantage point, you may become aware of certain life patterns you have created over time.

The brightly colored reddish-orange bracts of the Indian Paintbrush give off a highly artistic and passionate energy. By sitting with this plant, or by taking in its essence, you may feel a sense of emergence, warmth, and vitality. You may choose to take in this energy as a way to help you support your own needs for survival and to help you eliminate any parasitic relationships you may have with others. Indian Paintbrush may increase your awareness of any relationship in which one person is too dependent upon another. It may also bring to your awareness the times in your life when others have helped you survive and thrive.

Each of the chakras is also associated with a color. The movement, light, color, frequency, and vibration of each energy center influence your relationship to each energy center and to yourself as a whole person.

People have appreciated and responded to different colors since the beginning of time. You choose certain colors for the clothes you wear, the paint on your walls, your furniture, living room curtains, bath towels, kitchen wares, car, and even the foods you eat. We are surrounded by color. By becoming familiar with colors that are associated with the spectrum of the rainbow and the chakra energy centers of the body, you will begin to notice some very basic things about plants, nature, colors, and yourself. For example, when we pay attention, it seems natural for plants that are in the red, orange, and yellow color range to exude a warm, stimulating, and vibrant energy. They generally appear to be more connected to the earth and to our personality self—to our roots, our emotions, and our thoughts. You can actually feel this resonance as you look at them. The flowers in the blue and purple spectrums seem to be more connected to the sky. When you look at these flowers and pay attention to their colors, it stimulates a sense of inspiration, insight, vision, and clarity. These colors are cooling, like a breath of fresh air, and seem to take you to a deeper place of self-reflection based on intuition and insight. The pink color associated with the heart rests in between both; it engenders feelings of a mildly warm place. These colors are very soothing to the heart. The color white, associated with the energy center on the top of the head, gives a sense of purity, cleanliness, sacredness, and connectedness.

By no means do you have to be expert at understanding chakras to work with the flower cards. But you might want to think about the energy centers within your body, as well as the colors associated with them, as you begin to experience the wisdom of the flowers. It will deepen your experience of these gifts from Nature's bounty.

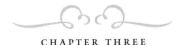

CHAPTER THREE

How to Use the Voices of Flowers Cards

The Voices of Flowers cards that accompany this book offer us another way of learning the messages from the plants and flowers. They can be a wonderful tool for self-reflection and self-discovery, helping you plant new seeds of awareness and open new doorways within yourself.

In this chapter I will suggest several different ways to use the cards, but I also invite you to find your own best ways of working with them.

Working with the cards should be a sacred and ceremonial experience. When I do a flower card reading, I like to create a relaxing and pleasant environment first. I usually do these readings either sitting or lying down to free the feeling of clutter in my mind, sometimes spreading a blanket outside if the weather allows. I keep a special cloth to spread the cards on and light candles to bring a feeling of peace. I recommend that you find a place where you can get quiet and create some sacred space. If you are in the middle of a busy day and do not have the time to create your preferred space, then prepare the space in your mind through visualization and imagination. What's important is not the particulars of your setting, only your ability to find a quiet place where you won't be interrupted and your intent to create some sacred space for the wisdom of the flowers to speak to you.

Through this ceremonial relationship with the flower cards, you will be able to access the wisdom of flowers and plants. The more you work with the cards, the more deeply you will come to understand how the flowers and their colors and qualities relate to your whole being. And the deeper you will come into relationship with your body.

Using liquid flower essences during your readings can enhance your experience of the different vibrations of the flowers. Of course, you will still receive tremendous benefit using the flower card deck on its own, but if you choose to enhance your practice by using the essences, you will find information about how to work with them on page 102 and how to order my Living Flower Essences in the Resources section.

THE BASICS OF A FLOWER CARD READING

When you are ready to use the cards, prepare your space and begin by asking yourself, *What is my intent? What is my presenting issue? What message from these magical flowers would serve me now?* If you don't have any special concerns in the moment, you can simply be in the silence of your mind.

Now take a look at the card deck. You'll see that each card shows a flower and its primary quality, which is the basic attribute of the flower. Study each card one by one. As you choose a card, notice how it relates to your own energy patterns. Look at the picture of the flower and notice its colors and personality. Notice how the flowers express themselves and pay attention to which flowers you are attracted to. The flowers, their colors, and their messages will help to stimulate your entire energy system. Read about the flower's primary quality and allow yourself to capture a sense of that quality. Take that feeling deep inside yourself.

Choose one or two cards that you are especially attracted to and look them up in the book. Read the Voice of the Flower and the Insight associated with that card or cards. Imagine the flower talking to you. You may want to read out loud, then close your eyes and listen to the wisdom of the flower with your heart. Take several minutes to allow yourself to take in the flower's message. If you are using flower essences, take three or four drops of the flowers you are studying before you read about them. Take in the experience and pay attention to subtle energy or emotional changes you may experience.

You may choose to work with one flower for several days or longer. Remember you have the freedom to choose any flower, any time. Follow your heart's desire. You will find similarities among the flowers and the affirmations. Through conscious repetition, the power of words and thoughts will become seeded in your memory. This allows you to manifest a state of consciousness that can alter your life forever. The flowers, as all of life, come from one source. Trust your process.

Another wonderful approach is to share a card reading with a friend or to choose a particular card spread with your partner. When you pair up with another, you can either create an intent together or work with separate intents.

If you aren't drawn to one particular card, you can also choose a card from a shuffled deck. After you shuffle the cards, simply lay them face down and choose a card drawing on your own intuition. I like to try to feel the energy of the cards when I do this. I place them in a circle and lightly place my hands above the cards and without touching them, rotating my hands clockwise. I then choose a card by its energy. Be assured that the magic of the cards will attract you to the exact message you need at the time.

You can also take your reading further by reading the Energy Impact or chakra correspondence for the flower you choose. (You can read more about the seven chakras on page 91.) Note which chakra energy centers are affected by the plant. Then read the Affirmations for the flower you are studying. Read them one at a time. Repeat each one aloud. If you like, you can write down the Affirmation and carry it with you, or place it on a mirror or in a special spot where you will be reminded of it throughout the day. Use the Affirmations as often as you wish throughout the day and before you go to bed. If you are working with essences, take a drop of the essence as you repeat the Affirmation.

USING THE CARDS FOR DAILY INSIGHT

Another way to use the Voices of Flowers cards is as a daily meditation tool. Ideally you would go to your sacred space for a few moments each day, some-place where you can listen to your heart. Then simply choose a card and let it be your guide for the day. Carefully look at the picture of the flower and its primary quality, and then place it in front of you. If you have the flower essence for that flower, take a few drops. Then close your eyes and imagine the energy and color of the flower embracing you and filling you. If you are focusing on healing a particular issue that relates to a certain chakra, bring the energy and color of your chosen flower into that energy center in your body. Let yourself be imbued by the presence of the flower as fully as possible. Then open your eyes and remember this experience throughout the day, holding the flower's message in your heart.

There is no one right way to use the cards. Try out some of the readings or the daily meditation or experiment with ways you like best. No matter how you use the cards, by using them regularly you will soon discover that a profound relationship is being created between the plants and flowers and yourself, a relationship that will take you on an incredible journey of self-exploration and discovery. Allow the flowers to grace you with their beauty, wisdom, and power. Let them nurture and embrace you with their light-filled energies. And remember, just as all seeds grow with tender loving care and guidance, by allowing the flowers to nourish and guide you, you too will blossom into your fullest expression of Self.

CHAPTER FOUR

Card Spreads

In the pages that follow, I offer four different spreads for you to choose from: The Flower Spread, The Seed Spread, The Four Elements/Circle of Life Spread, and The Chakra Card Spread. Before you choose which one to use, I recommend that you review them all and closely observe your response to each one. Go with the one that really calls out to you.

Once you have determined which card spread you are most drawn to, take some time to silence your mind and follow the suggestions made in chapter three for identifying your intent. Remember this is a process of joining the flower spirits in the nature realm and calling upon them for help.

LAYING OUT THE CARDS

Laying out a spread should be a ceremonial process in itself. No matter which spread you choose, always take a few moments to get comfortable and focus yourself, then shuffle the cards and lay them face down in a circle. (You can also simply choose the cards from a face-down deck.)

Staying focused on your intent, pick up the card you are most drawn to, turn it over, and look at it. Observe any responses you may have to your chosen card, then place the card face up. As you choose a card for each position in a particular layout, be aware of the position of the card and remain focused on your intent.

When you have completed the layout, all the cards you have selected should be face up and placed in their given positions in the spread. Take a moment to look at each card, then read the cards one by one, starting with the one in the first position. Go back to the book and look up its Voice, its Insight, its Energy Impact, and its Affirmations. Notice any feelings or thoughts or images that come to you as you experience each flower card and its specific position in the spread.

After you have read the last card in your spread, go back and try to gain a perspective of the whole reading. Look at all the cards together and see what they say to you. Let yourself be guided intuitively to any place or position within the card layout that particularly calls to you. Let the cards tell your story.

If you'd like, you may ask yourself questions such as, *Which card/s am I most drawn to? Where in the reading does the most energy show up for me? In what way has this reading opened my awareness about myself, my situation, or my intent?*

Notice any significant or possibly even hidden messages in the reading. What was the most meaningful to you? What have you gained from considering the whole picture of your card layout? What was the overall message given to you?

Always, as you come to completion with a given card layout, give thanks to the flowers and their messages. Let yourself absorb the reading as your story unfolds.

THE FLOWER SPREAD

This spread teaches you about your inherent connection with Mother Earth and Father Sky. It will awaken your awareness and encourage you to tend to the flowering of yourself. The messages of this spread will strengthen your personal power and understanding of yourself, providing guidance and support. It will help you achieve a higher perspective on your life's situation and give new meaning to your life choices.

For this spread, the cards are laid out as follows:

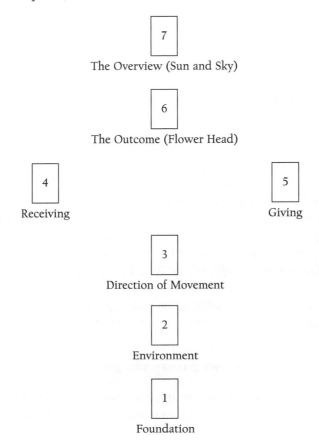

The Cards and What They Symbolize

Card Position One: Foundation (Root)

This card represents the foundation of your present situation or current relationship to yourself. Your foundation is also associated with the root energy center that connects you to the Earth and serves as your grounding energy. The Foundation card takes you to the root of your question or to the foundation of your quest. It points you toward the strength of your foundation. It may indicate what is happening in your life on a deeper or unconscious level that has not yet been brought forth, such as in your dreams, buried emotions, memories, desires, and thoughts. The root card will help you gain an awareness of your relationship to the source of the situation.

Card Position Two: Environment (Earth)

The card in the second position relates to the soil or the type of environment that you are providing for yourself in which to grow. The message of this card calls upon you to get in touch with your style of living and your personality self to see how you care for your root energies.

Are you providing a rich, nurturing environment? One that is well-watered and well-tended? Or have you neglected your environment? The flower you draw will reveal what is the most nurturing environmental energies for your intention or desire. This message will also teach you a deeper understanding of how the environment of your thoughts, emotions, and attitudes affects your roots.

Card Position Three: Direction of Movement (Stem)

The Direction of Movement card speaks to you of the energies that move through you and motivate you. What inspires you to make choices and take new directions in life? What draws you to the actions you take? Do the choices that you make reflect your inner environment and the root energies in which you reside? The message of this card tells you more about your process and how it is working for you, and it offers insight into what direction your movement should take. The truths of this card will deepen your awareness of how to nurture your growth, how to make better choices, and how to find the next step on your path.

Card Position Four: Receiving (Left Leaf)

The Receiving card relates to circumstances both outside and within yourself. This card indicates the energies you are taking in, what you are breathing into your being, how you are receiving these energies, and in what way you are internalizing them. What is your psychic space and how is it feeding the situation? This card speaks of receiving Higher Wisdom and filling the branches of your creativity and inspirations to build upon your roots, environment, and the direction of movement you choose to take. It is about receiving your gifts, talents, and abilities and nurturing them.

Card Position Five: Giving (Right Leaf)

The Giving card also relates to circumstances both outside and within yourself. This card indicates the energies you are giving out, what you are exhaling and releasing. The Giving card speaks to you of the way you express and balance yourself in the world and allows you to let go of that which holds you back. Your direction is becoming clearer, your creativity stronger, and through your own nourishment of self, you feel yourself growing in ways that not only feed yourself but also feed others.

Card Position Six: The Outcome (Flower Head)

The Outcome card resembles the blossoming flower at its fullest. The message of this card is a revelation of what you will achieve. It assures you that you have the freedom and innate capacity to reach your fullest exaltation, to express your core essence. This card speaks to you of emergence. It offers a natural resolution, completion, and understanding of the outcome of the reading.

Card Position Seven: The Overview (Sun and Sky)

The Overview card is associated with higher consciousness and Divine wisdom. It indicates how to align yourself with your spiritual essence and intrinsic knowing deep inside. The Overview gives the perspective of wisdom and the healing power of grace to the outcome. The flower head blooms and fades, but the Sun and Sky remain.

This card honors what is sacred in your heart, allowing that which is in your heart to connect to your higher wisdom. See, feel, and experience yourself as a vibrant and whole being.

RENEWAL—THE SEED SPREAD

You may have come to a time in your life when you realize how worn out you feel, how tired you are of certain patterns in your life, and how much you are in need of a retreat or change in your life. You may be looking forward to time out from your mundane responsibilities, or you may yearn to be in silence. If you are feeling these things, you may be in need of a renewal. Renewal is a natural part of a continuous process of cleansing, building, and creating. Renewal is about taking time to consciously release old habits of mind and body that are no longer desired or needed. Letting go of burdens brings a fresh beginning. Taking time to be with yourself helps you to let go and relax. The cards you choose in The Seed Spread can empower your process of renewal and rekindle your relationship with yourself.

In the Seed Spread you will choose four flower cards. The first card, Planting, is the seed you are sowing. The second card, Nurturing, is the quality or direction of its growth. The third card, Unfolding, is the fullness of its blossom. The final or fourth card is Harvesting, or the nature of the fruit that will be born. They are laid out in a horizontal line, as follows:

17

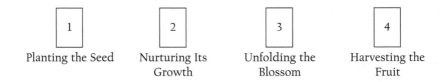

1	2	3	4
Planting the Seed	Nurturing Its Growth	Unfolding the Blossom	Harvesting the Fruit

Card Position One: Planting the Seed

Before you choose your first card for the Seed Spread, take a moment to reflect on how you've been feeling and get in touch with ways you may not feel connected with yourself. The card you choose at this time is about acknowledging your need for change and healing. Gently bring your focus to that silent, powerful place at the center of your being. Allow the silence in this sacred place to envelop you. When you feel ready, choose a card. Let the card bring to your awareness an energy that can help you with your renewal. Contemplate the image of the flower, the flower's message, insight, and affirmations. Rest in the source of your renewal.

Card Position Two: Nurturing Its Growth

When you choose your second card for the Seed Spread, ask for guidance from the flowers for an energy that supports, nurtures, and gives you life. Allow the flower to help you grow this renewing energy, awakening the bud of new life within you. Let your thoughts and images of this flower card share its qualities with you, and notice how this flower nurtures and supports you. Listen to your inner voice. Let the soil for your seed (your inner environment) be tended and cared for as you experience an expansion in your awareness. As you nurture and renew yourself, the seed opens further and begins to grow.

Card Position Three: Unfolding the Blossom

When you choose your third card for the Seed Spread, you may be feeling a sense of renewal dawning. Let this card help your renewal to unfold. Choose a card and notice how the flower helps you feel uplifted and reconnected within. Read the flower's voice and hear its words. Listen to its message and contemplate its energy. Let your inner being come forth and embrace the feeling of freedom and renewal. Allow yourself to blossom to your fullest, feeling refreshed, whole, and at peace with yourself.

Card Position Four: Harvesting the Fruit

When you choose the final card of this spread, it is now time to celebrate the fruition of your growth. The seed has opened, the sprout has grown, the bud has formed, and the blossom has bloomed. You are now ready for the harvest. Having been gifted with new awareness and understanding, welcome and honor your renewal by sharing your bounty with others. Joyfully yield the abundant harvest of your fruits.

THE FOUR ELEMENTS CIRCLE OF LIFE SPREAD

For this spread, each of the four elements is placed in connection to its direction—Earth in the North direction, Fire in the South, Air in the East, and Water in the West, forming a complete circle, just as if you were looking at a map of the world, with the addition of the elements.

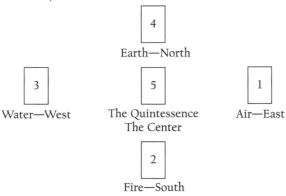

In the center of the four elements is the "Quintessence" card, which represents an invisible energy source that can be felt and experienced as an expression of the seed of the universe, the core essence, and the Divine Presence of all living things. As a whole, the four elements and the "Quintessence" produce a powerful and effective means of healing.

The elements, including the blossoming flower, for example, are what create a flower essence. The core essence of the flower is considered the "Quintessence." The elements of Air, Fire, Water, and Earth are living foods that sustain and nurture us. They support all of life and give us everything that we need.

Using this spread allows you to experience and understand your relationship to each of the elements including your "quintessence." It will help you experience an overview or a higher perspective about your life's situation and will take you to a deeper connection with and understanding of your core or the very essence of your being.

Various cultures and people have different associations with the elements and the four directions. This card spread is based more on the European Celtic associations. The attributes, images, elements, and colors correlated with any given direction may differ from culture to culture or path to path.

Card Position One: Air—East
This card is represented by the direction East and the Air in which we live and breathe. Just as the sun rises, bringing forth a new day of illumination and power, we are given a new hope, energized by the Light, allowing ourselves to perceive from a place that expands beyond our physical world. As the eagle soars, we can see below us yet be connected to our earthly ways. As springtime emerges, new buds and plant growth bring freshness and beauty adorning the earth with living color and natural bounty.

We are sustained by the oxygen provided by plants and trees. Without them, we could not survive. The East represents new beginnings, new life budding, and inspiration. As you take in a new breath of fresh air, imagine yourself taking in the green bounty of plant energy deep inside your throat and lungs. Breathe in the wisdom of this card's message and allow it to move through your entire being. In this place, you will be given clarity. You may decide upon a new idea or project to work on, or a door may open in some way that gives you a new insight about yourself or about a situation you are in. You may be guided to speak your truths, sing your songs, and listen to your sounds and vibrations.

Card Position Two: Fire—South

This card is represented by the direction South and the Fire or Sun which gives us the source of energy that provides light and heat. It is sunlight which makes possible the process of photosynthesis, especially in plants, where the synthesis of complex organic materials such as carbohydrates from carbon dioxide, water, and inorganic salts, with the aid of a catalyst such as chlorophyll, gives us an enrichment of vitamins and minerals. The South card is associated with your personal growth and the fire or inner light within your body. The message of this card may call upon you get to know yourself, to look at the ways you reason and think, to find your purpose and desires in life, and to empower yourself to be who you need to be. The power of the South and the Sun gives you the courage and faith to act upon and trust your intuition and innocence. It strengthens you to live life in joy and humor and to trust your childlike self. By doing so and by loving yourself, you develop honor, dignity, and self-esteem.

Choosing this card gives you the opportunity to allow your creativity to come through, to develop your ideas, and to trust the power of your thoughts and your intuition.

Card Position Three: Water—West

This card represents the direction West and the element Water. The flowing action of water creates movement and change upon the earth. Its patterns change the earth's appearance. Water feeds the earth, without it, the earth would become barren and unable to produce plants, trees, and flowers. Water sustains us by stabilizing our bodies internally: aiding us in the process of elimination and detoxification of the body, managing blood pressure, and preserving cellular efficiency.

Water is related to our emotional center and is the driving force which gives us the incentive and the creativity to get where we want to go and to help us get in touch with how we feel. When our emotions become stagnant and there is no flow, we shut down and become suppressed. Our thoughts become dry and negative, and our hearts become closed. A steady flow of water within the body can penetrate negativity, nourishing us, and fertilizing our thoughts with healing power. When we feel this flow of loving, our hearts reopen, and we are able to give back love to others.

The direction of West is also symbolic of taking a retreat or of going within. Taking time for ourselves through introspection, especially before making decisions, allows us to be present and to feel from the inside before acting on the outside. A renewed self-expression and creativity will keep us flowing and moving, offering a rebirth in how we pursue our purpose.

Card Position Four : Earth—North

This card represents the direction North and the element Earth, whereby all living things are provided with sustenance and nourishment. The power of North is a time of renewal, purity, and quickening of the spirit. Although the earth appears dormant and barren in the cold and windy winters of the North, the seeds of inner reflection become active. A breath of spiritual renewal takes place in the midst of the cooling winds. The North card reflects a time of gathering strength, becoming clear with your intent, and finding resources upon the earth to bring forth into your life.

The North is the place of the elders from which wisdom is offered in how to live in harmony with the earth such as toolmaking, building shelter, and cultivating. The message of Earth is associated with our relationship to the material world and our ability to survive. The plants and trees of the earth provide us with food, shelter, clothing, and medicine.

Through natural laws we learn how to navigate in the material world, grounding our energy in ways that connect us to the earth, building our foundation for how we live out our lives. Our relationship to the material world impacts our life force energy and the ways in which we breathe and move. The message of this card gives us wisdom, harmony, and support in the ways we are inspired to create in the world. The earth offers us an abundance of resources, both inner and outer. As we honor and respect her, we will come to honor and respect ourselves and all of Creation. The message here is to honor where we came from, who we are, what we are becoming, and to express gratitude for all living things.

Card Position Five: The Quintessence—The Center

This card is represented as the very core essence of your being, by the Divine Presence that is already inherently within you. This is your sacred center, the place where you can always go for prayer, meditation, and connection with your deepest sense of Self.

The Quintessence shows you that you are an expression of the Divine Source that lives and breathes through you. This is the place that aligns you with your Higher Power, giving you wisdom and spiritual insight. The message of this card is to remind you to go to your Higher Source, your sacred space, the place that gives you personal freedom and expression. In this place, you will come to an understanding that all living things are interdependent upon each other. You will soon discover how your own personal essence integrates, receives, and gives back to the seed essence of the universe. The message of this card will teach you your role in the Circle of Life. If you wander from this place, remember this is only an illusion. For wherever you are, whatever you're doing, the sacred center is only a breath away.

THE CHAKRA CARD SPREAD

Begin this card reading by setting an intent for your path of healing. This spread is about listening to the voices and messages of the flowers that connect with the energy centers or chakras within your body. Remember that each energy center or chakra resonates with each other, integrating and mirroring who you are. You may wish to read chapter two and the Going Deeper section on page 91 for more information about the chakras.

If your intent, for example, is to gain insight about a particular health issue and how that issue affects your whole being, begin by shuffling the cards and choosing a card one by one for each chakra, keeping your focus clear.

Some flower cards may naturally be associated with the chakra energy center you are working with. Some may not. Don't be concerned about the color of the flower or that it needs to correspond with the color of the chakra. In this spread you are receiving insights from any of the flowers in relationship to any of the chakras. Let's say you choose the Blue Flag Iris card for the first chakra regarding a health issue. If you read about Blue Flag, you will know the message is about stamina and pacing yourself. Perhaps the Blue Flag will give you inspirations or an insight into how you can better pace yourself and avoid the burnout that is reflected through your physical body and the health issue that you have.

Or maybe you will choose Black-Eyed Susan to represent the fourth chakra. Although the colors of the Black-Eyed Susan are not associated with the colors of the fourth chakra, the message and the voice of Black-Eyed Susan may bring to your awareness the ways in which you shut down your heart and feel challenged to love.

The layout of the Chakra Spread is very straightforward. You'll simply create a vertical line, with the first card at the bottom and the seventh card at the top, as follows:

| 7 |

The Crown or Seventh Chakra

| 6 |

The Third Eye, Ajna, Brow, or Sixth Chakra

| 5 |

Throat or Fifth Chakra

| 4 |

Heart or Fourth Chakra

| 3 |

Mental, Solar Plexus, or Third Chakra

| 2 |

Emotional, Spleen, or Second Chakra

| 1 |

Root Energy or First Chakra

Card Position One: Root Energy or First Chakra

When you choose a flower card to reflect upon your relationship with your root or first chakra, you are focusing on your physical connection with yourself and with the earth. It may bring to you an awareness of the physical ways in which you survive, such as the food you eat, the amount of exercise you do, where you live, where you work, and the physical environments you choose to be in. The root chakra is also the center of primal energy, it reflects your spiritual and soul heritage—where you came from and how that has affected who you are now, and where you want to go now. Whether your parents were poor, middle class, or wealthy, the way that you connect to your material survival as a child and as an adult may not be the same. Beneath the surface of this kind of survival is the survival and relationship to yourself, your life force energy, and the way you breathe and move with the earth.

Card Position Two: Emotional, Spleen, or Second Chakra

When you choose a flower card to give you insight into your relationship with your second chakra, your intent is related to your emotions. You may want some deeper insight into how you flow with the emotional current within, or how you express yourself creatively. You may also feel the flow of your expression as a sexual, sensual, and passionate being. Perhaps you will gain some insight into the deeper currents within that affect the flow of your overall emotional health. Drink plenty of water and eat good nutrients, letting the flow within you spread, move, and come alive!

Card Position Three: Mental, Solar Plexus, or Third Chakra

When you choose a flower card to reflect upon your relationship with the third chakra, you are inviting introspection into the way that you think and view yourself. You will begin to notice how your thoughts—positive or negative—feed your emotional body and how you walk on this earth. You may learn to think and perceive in clearer ways without judgment and criticism. The flower card that you receive at this time may bring insight to your dignity, values, desires, thoughts, and will. Perhaps you will be guided to align with the Divine will, trusting your intuition and your knowledge.

Card Position Four: Heart or Fourth Chakra

When you choose a flower card for insight about your relationship with the fourth chakra, you may be coming to a deeper understanding of the value of forgiveness, of letting go, of learning to live and feel what it is to love unconditionally. As your heart becomes more open, you may feel an extension of warmth radiating outward, and you may find yourself becoming more tolerant and generous toward yourself and others. A doorway to your path of healing is opening wider, and you are allowing yourself to let your heart guide you in the choices you make.

Card Position Five: Throat or Fifth Chakra

When you choose a flower card for insight into your relationship with your throat or fifth chakra, bring your awareness to your throat area and feel the vibrations of the sounds that you make. Remember that the expression of communication is the passage of our inner selves to the outside world and the responses that are returned to us. Our inner self includes the sounds and vibrations of our voice, our thoughts, inner truths, and insights. Notice the way that you communicate with the words you choose and the tones you make. Are you listening to your heart when you speak to others? Are you listening to the ways that others communicate to you? Perhaps there are other creative forms of expression such as dance, sculpture, painting, singing, sound, chanting, writing, playing instruments, which would fulfill your expression for life.

Card Position Six: Third Eye, Ajna, Brow, or Sixth Chakra

When you choose a flower card for insight into the sixth chakra, you may be gaining a deeper understanding of trusting your perception, your intuition, and the way you view the world from a higher perspective. You may be forming a new relationship with the Higher Power that is already inherently within you, feeling an opening in your psychic awareness and the ability to see beyond time and space. Perhaps you will receive a broader vision, an expanded view of your intent for this card spread. You may experience a deeper understanding of your intent, allowing the power of illumination to come forth.

Card Position Seven: The Crown or Seventh Chakra

When you choose a flower card for insight into your relationship with the seventh chakra, you may be comforted to know that you are connected with and part of an all-inclusive Presence where there is no separation. Although at times you may feel alone in the circumstances that you face in life, you must know on some level, that someone else somewhere is experiencing something very similar to yourself. You come to realize that all of humankind and all life-forms on this earth are part of a bigger picture and that we are all in this together.

As you gain access to the energy field of the crown chakra, you become aligned with a Higher Power that is linked to the higher consciousness of all. Perhaps your connection with the crown chakra will open a new way to how you view yourself, the intent of this card reading, and the way that you interact in the world. You may feel a vibrant energy flow throughout your body, emotions, mind, and heart and open up your ability to see beyond your wildest imagination.

CHAPTER FIVE

The Flowers: Aster to Yucca

The wisdom contained in flowers is subtle and ever changing, yet there are specific qualities and energies that you can discover as you begin your study of flowers and their essences and work with the Voices of Flowers cards. Whether you occasionally choose a card, use them as a daily meditation tool, or try the various spreads, this is the chapter you will want to turn to read about the flowers you choose.

The flowers are listed in alphabetical order. For each one, you will find a Primary Quality, Voice, Insight, Energy Impact, and Affirmation. Explore the flowers, listen to their voices, and develop your own relationships with these vibrant living and life-giving plants. As you invite the Voices of Flowers into your life through your work with the cards, let the spirit of the flowers guide you and help you to discover the depths of your innermost mysteries.

ASTER

(Machaeranthera tephrodes)
PRIMARY QUALITY: ILLUMINATION

Voice of the Flower

"The radiant yellow glow from within the center of my eye shines forth to you. Feel its warmth, and let light in. Like a shining star, I am guiding you to turn toward the brightness of your own illumination. As you fill yourself with light, you will feel an opening in your mind's eye. Let your intuition and higher vision expand as my purple rays radiate outward to begin a new path of natural evolution. Come fully into the presence of this moment, guided by your intuition, connected with yourself.

"Share your visions and understanding with children and hold them in love and light."

Insight

When you choose the Aster card, you are inviting illumination and insight to guide you on your path of personal growth and spiritual evolution. Aster offers balance and inspiration through vision and wisdom, allowing you to see more deeply from within. Perhaps Aster is giving you an opportunity to embrace a greater community awareness and to follow through on higher spiritual principles of living and being in the world. You may be inspired to participate in a community project related to environmental protection, water conservation, animal rights, or activities for children and teens. Share these inspirations with the children and give them light and love.

Energy Impact (chakra correspondence)
3rd, 6th, and 7th chakras

Affirmations

"I see the deeper meaning behind all life situations and act from a place of wisdom and insight."

"May light flow within me and all around me and guide me to my highest good."

"I accept all that is and will be. My future is bright before me and the path easy to find. I trust my intuition and I am my own shining star."

BELLS-OF-IRELAND

(Moluccella laevis)

PRIMARY QUALITY: INNER-CHILD TRANSFORMATION

Voice of the Flower

"Welcome to my Nature Kingdom. I offer you protection in my inner sanctuary. You will feel a deep silence and security here along with a magical presence of my plant's Nature Spirits. Allow yourself to be nurtured and guided by the Nature Spirits. Communicate and connect with them. Hold the power of their gentle presence in your heart and trust their strength. By doing so, you will feel a deep sense of strength rise within yourself, and your heart will fill with love. Let love pour through your heart and heal your inner child and the children of the world."

Insight

When you choose the Bells-of-Ireland card, your path of healing is calling you to seek a secure and nurturing environment. Bells-of-Ireland guide you to connect with Nature Spirits, to take time to create an opportunity to sit in a garden, or under a tree, or simply to find a safe and quiet place to be. Allow yourself to open, yield, and be guided by your natural instincts. Find the strength needed to gently act upon these instincts and to trust them. Perhaps this is a time to explore inner-child issues and to cleanse emotional wounds of the heart.

Energy Impact (chakra correspondence)
4th and 7th chakras

Affirmations
"I give myself the freedom to express vulnerability and trust in a safe and
  nurturing environment."

"I am drawn to those of like minds who nurture, love, and protect my
  friendship with them."

"I let love pour through my heart and heal my inner child."

BLACK-EYED SUSAN

(Rudbeckia hirta)
PRIMARY QUALITY: INNER PEACE

Voice of the Flower
"I invite you to enter the darkness of my inner circle, and feel the shadow
within my core. Allow your own shadow to merge with mine in this void.
Experience your awareness of this void without judgment, as you stretch outward toward the rays of my golden halo. Feeling the warmth and radiance of
my halo, fill your body-mind-soul with that which gives you peace and light.
Permeate your thoughts with the power of being free, whole, and at peace
with yourself. And in this place, experience peace within."

Insight
When you choose the Black-Eyed Susan card, you may be on a path of healing where you are being asked to face your shadow self. By accepting and
embracing any darkness you may feel, you can then release it to your Higher
Source. By trusting in the mystery of your darkness, perhaps you will expe-

rience a positive role that darkness brings to your personal awareness and growth. Black-Eyed Susan helps you heal by understanding who you are now, finding purpose and hope in yourself and your life circumstances. As you experience the liberating principle of this plant, inner peace awaits you.

Energy Impact (chakra correspondence)
1st, 3rd, and 7th chakras

Affirmations
"I give myself permission to embrace my pains and to release them to God so that I may feel inner peace."

"I am willing to be transformed, restored, and rejuvenated and to claim all parts of who I am."

"I am free and whole. I have the power to believe in myself and to feel at peace with who I am."

"May I stir the power within me to create loving and peaceful thoughts."

BLANKETFLOWER

(Gaillardia pulchella)
PRIMARY QUALITY: FIRE DANCE

Voice of the Flower
"I attract those who seek pleasure in living, and I invite you to step inside my vibrant colors. Feel my warmth and exuberance. Let yourself experience the sensations and radiance of my vibrant presence. May my joyful and creative expression arouse your vital life force energy and move even the tiniest cells in your body-mind-soul. Let me stir your passion for living. Dance yourself into a newfound freedom of thought, emotion, and action. May the light within you come alive!"

Insight

When you choose the Blanketflower card, you are being reminded to embrace the radiance within you, to kick off your shoes and feel the freedom to take new steps in the dance of life. Blanketflower offers a fun-loving attitude and the willingness to choose the brighter side. It teaches you the power of your emotions and the energetic impact they have upon your life. It empowers your thoughts with a purpose in life that is guided by your higher Will. So go have fun! Create a new project. Do something that fills you up and gives you life!

Energy Impact (chakra correspondence)

1st, 2nd, and 3rd chakras

Affirmations

"I am a sacred flame of the Divine, dancing with joy and celebrating life."

"Passionate consuming flames burn away all my fears."

"May I arouse the fire within me to move forth in life with warmth and exuberance."

34

BLUE FLAG IRIS

(Iris missouriensis)
PRIMARY QUALITY: STAMINA

Voice of the Flower

"Although I may be challenged by the barriers that present themselves to me, my growth continues at a slow and steady pace. I have learned that skillful pacing of my life's journey helps me to build stamina and endurance when facing hardships or stress. From beneath the bog, I am able to rise above any preconceived limitations and self-centered aspects of myself (including the mundane, the material, and the world's inflictions), with the realization that the Divine in me is an infinite resource and the prime doer. I am inspired by the beauty of Divine grace and Divine timing. My subtle rainbow colors build a bridge that brings together any disharmony, uplifting me toward greater aspirations of creativity, simplicity, and imagination. Receive my gifts. You, too, can rise from the bog."

Insight

When you choose the Blue Flag Iris card, it is reminding you to slow down and pace yourself in order to build stamina and to prevent burnout. In what way are you feeling stuck in the bog? In what ways do you lack inspiration or creativity to help find your way out? Blue Flag Iris draws you upward, directing you to rise above the material, mundane, and self-imposed limitations you have of yourself by helping you see and experience the Divine within you as your true Source, appreciating the beauty that comes from within. This card serves as an inspiration, attracting the colors of the rainbow and making a bridge between what enters and leaves you. Perhaps this is a good time to give thought to new insights about yourself or to feel inspired to write, paint, and/or to express your artistic talent in some creative way.

Energy Impact (chakra correspondence)

3rd, 5th, 6th, and 7th chakras

Affirmations

"I face life's setbacks with creativity and inspiration to spiral upward."

"I trust that my perseverance and stamina will help me get through any healing crisis that I need to encounter."

"I fully embrace my inner beauty and integrity in the perfect image of my Divine being."

"As the Creator is the prime doer, I trust all is being Divinely orchestrated."

BOUNCING BET

(Saponaria officinalis)

PRIMARY QUALITY: MYSTIC UNION

Voice of the Flower

"I am the power of love within you singing deep into your heart. My compassion and bliss harmonize the Divine union of the opposites within yourself as well as with your beloved. This Divine union is the union of self with Self. As you feel the wholeness of love within yourself, you are more capable of unconditionally loving another. It takes a great love to love yourself and your beloved without interfering with the natural laws of human nature. Allow the mystery of your union to unfold, accepting imperfections, yet changing conditions so that there is greater harmony and love within yourself and with your beloved."

Insight

Bouncing Bet brings to your awareness the sacred inner marriage within yourself. Offering receptivity, openness, and union of self with Self (lower and higher self), Bouncing Bet helps you to receive and give love. This flower allows you to appreciate the mystery of who you are and to find ways that bring harmony to your home and heart. Take some time to reflect, asking yourself, *In what ways do I love and take care of myself? What experiences in my life give me love and help me feel loving? How do I give love back?* Observe your thoughts, feelings, and any body awareness as you reflect upon your responses.

Energy Impact *(chakra correspondence)*

1st, 4th, and 7th chakras

Affirmations

"I am the power of love singing deep into my heart."

"I awaken the love in my heart to fulfill my most intimate passions."

"Let the doorway of my heart open wide for love to flow freely through me."

CALENDULA

(Calendula officinalis)
PRIMARY QUALITY: CALM

Voice of the Flower
"I bring to you a softness that will quiet your mind and emotions and will fill you with the radiance of my gentle presence. My soothing orange and yellow light will warm your inner world and nurture that place inside that yearns for peace. In this state of calmness you will become more aware of your thoughts and feelings, releasing any negativity you may have toward yourself or others. May you gain the inner confidence to trust in yourself and make choices that bring to you a sense of inner peace and calm."

Insight
When you choose the Calendula card, ask yourself, *What circumstances in life cause me to feel nervous and tense? What can I do to bring more calmness to myself and to my life circumstances?* Calendula calms nervousness and anxious emotions, bringing a quiet centering to the abdomen and solar plexus area. Calendula provides an inner warmth and radiance that promotes sensitivity and understanding in the way you relate to yourself and others. Perhaps Calendula beckons you to do something soothing for yourself such as to take a relaxing bath or sit by a sunny window or read a good book.

Energy Impact (chakra correspondence)
2nd and 3rd chakras

Affirmations
"I fill myself with a gentle glow of orange and yellow light."
"I allow peaceful, easy emotions to emerge and be felt."
"I create positive, calm, and thoughtful energy."

37

CALIFORNIA POPPY

(Eschscholtzia californica)

PRIMARY QUALITY: PURIFIER

Voice of the Flower

"Let me wrap myself around you and hold you inside my deep rich orange presence. Feel my protection. May the fiery glow of my petals give you insight into your thoughts and feelings, bringing to your awareness any emotional toxins that you carry. Surrender into my shielding embrace and allow your inner knowing to trust my process. As I slowly unfold my petals into the morning sunlight, may your thoughts and emotions be lifted. Let my gentle radiance encapsulate you. Feel the freedom as you cleanse."

Insight

When you choose the California Poppy card, your path of healing is to find ways to care for yourself emotionally. If you are feeling emotionally closed down in any way, California Poppy offers cleansing and purification of emotions or emotional patterns that no longer benefit you. Notice thoughts or feelings of anger, sadness, remorse, or other kinds of emotional toxins you feel you need to let go of. Be sure to isolate and identify each specific emotion. California Poppy can help you tap into your inner knowing of when to be receptive and open and when to protect your vulnerability. This is an opportunity to look at your emotional patterns without judgment. Allow yourself to experience an emotional release in some way.

Energy Impact (chakra correspondence)

2nd chakra

Affirmations

"I release my feelings of anger, fear, sadness, and shame and pray for emotional cleansing."

"I am the power of purification. May my thoughts and feelings be purified."

"I radiate light, wisdom, and love."

"I stir my passion and excitement for life and living."

CENTURY PLANT

(Agave parryi)

PRIMARY QUALITY: BREAKTHROUGH

Voice of the Flower

"Many seasons I have waited, in spring rains, in the long and hot desert sun, in winter frost and snow. And still I wait. The base of my spiny armor protects me from would-be predators for many years. I reach deep within my roots to provide for my long life and take each moment with care. My life is a journey of surrender and discovery while growing into my own strength. Slowly I emerge. In the midst of the silence of flourishing desert harmony, all of nature observes my bold and inescapable transformation. For it is in my rising glory in this final midsummer season that my sacred purpose is served and highest good prevails. I shudder not, nor do I recoil from this glory that finds its end. I bring to completion a deep connection with all. Surrendering with ease, quickly I go in totality, to prepare my seeds, a new birth, for another lifetime."

Insight

When you get the Century Plant card, it signifies that a breakthrough is on its way. Century Plant teaches courage, patience, strength, and survival as a natural process. By staying focused on your life goals and the ways you feed your strength and expression of yourself, you honor yourself. There may be something you need to let go of so you can move on. Perhaps it is time to embrace a new cycle of birth and celebration and decide what it is in your life that needs a breakthrough.

Energy Impact (chakra correspondence)
1st, 2nd, and 3rd chakras

Affirmations
"I am willing to let go of the old and become who I see myself to be."

"I take action for my own growth and changes."

"I am empowered through the Divine in me to be focused, creative, and to embrace my highest good."

"I am a vessel of the Divine, cocreating each moment."

CHAMOMILE (GERMAN)

(Matricaria chamomilla)
PRIMARY QUALITY: SERENITY

Voice of the Flower
"Come be with my cheerful nature and lightheartedness. I am here to help you feel brightness and joy, sharing your happiness with others. I give you comfort and remind you to slow down, relax, and be aware of the pleasant things of life that you enjoy. Take time to appreciate yourself and to find ways to relieve your tension and stress. My tranquil disposition offers you a serene way of living, giving you emotional balance and emotional stability."

Insight
Take time to sit, relax, and center yourself. Look at the Chamomile card and notice how it makes you feel. When you get the Chamomile card, you are being given an opportunity to evaluate your lifestyle and to change the ways you build tension and stress. You will find Chamomile to be uplifting, releasing tension and promoting peace and balance. If you have difficulty sleeping, are worried, or if you have a crying baby or irritable child, this card may be suggesting to drink Chamomile tea or to take a Chamomile flower essence.

Energy Impact (chakra correspondence)
3rd and 7th chakras

Affirmations
"I choose thoughts, feelings, and activities that comfort me emotionally."

"I take time out to relax and center myself."

"I release any anger, irritability, or impatience and seek serenity."

CHICORY

(Cichorium intybus)

PRIMARY QUALITY: INTERRELATEDNESS

Voice of the Flower
"I bring to you the gift of seeing yourself through the eyes of others, experiencing all life-forms as One with all of creation. May you use these gifts to awaken your awareness toward understanding natural laws. Through this understanding you open yourself to experience and respect heartfelt concern for others, honoring humanity and all earth life. We are all one family. Allow the doorway to open and trust your ability to love, respect, care for, and honor yourself and all your relations."

Insight
When you choose the Chicory card, you are being asked to go within yourself and connect with the core of your being that has feeling for yourself and others. If you have not been in harmony with yourself or with others, Chicory helps you to understand natural laws such as "what goes around, comes around." It offers the gift of heartfelt concern for others through genuine sharing in spite of differences. You may need to ask yourself who or what it is in your life that needs to experience unconditional love from you.

Energy Impact (chakra correspondence)
5th and 6th chakras

Affirmations
"We are all one in the circle of life."

"I honor, respect, and care for myself and all my relations."

"As I feel the expansion of my inner growth, I freely share this with others."

CLIFF ROSE

(Cowania mexicana)
PRIMARY QUALITY: POSITIVE SELF-IMAGE

Voice of the Flower
"Step inside my open petals and feel my gentle embrace. My fragrance is soft and sweet, and its presence will soothe your mind and body. I will bring you to your inner realms of awakening and help you value all that you are. My foundation is strong. I can grow between rocks and on dry earth. I have the power to show you your own strength and beauty. My healing presence is strong, yet humble. I attract only those who notice me and who desire to awaken to the true understanding of self-value and self-acceptance. Sip my nectar and feel the power of my love."

Insight
When you get the Cliff Rose card, you may be in need of a gentle, uplifting boost. There may be something within yourself that you are not accepting or valuing. You are being given an opportunity to look at and let go of your doubts and fears. Create an intent to work on a specific issue that you have with yourself which relates to your self-image, self-confidence, and your ability to love yourself. Begin in silence and take time to connect with what it is

that would help you feel more focused and positive about yourself. What is your relationship to yourself like? Do you do loving things for yourself? Do you take care of yourself? Cliff Rose awakens you to empower and love yourself and to be guided by your "higher good," creating a positive self-image. You might consider doing something special for yourself (or for your children) such as cooking a special dinner, making a favorite dessert, or going to see a movie.

Energy Impact (chakra correspondence)
3rd and 7th chakras

Affirmations
"I think well of myself and respect who I am as a child of the universe."
"My true image of Self is unblemished by the judgment of others."
"I release self-doubts and fears and allow myself to be who I am."

COLUMBINE (YELLOW)

(Aguilegia chrysantha)
PRIMARY QUALITY: DIVINE BEAUTY

Voice of the Flower
"My graceful elegance resonates with the golden treasure of Divine beauty from deep within. My light-filled vessel twinkles with cheer, goodness, and beauty for all. I will help you discover, nurture, and unveil your own sacred treasure of Divine beauty. Let go of any flawed images you may have about yourself, accepting and loving your true expression of beauty. Honor all of that which you are. Let your Divine beauty shine out for all to see, feel, hear, and touch. Receive all the goodness life has to offer you and give it back in the expression of your divine beauty. Embrace the Divine beauty in all of life and in every living thing."

Insight

When you choose the Columbine card, you may be unable to see your own inner worth and beauty. What is it that holds you back from seeing and feeling the beauty within yourself? What are you avoiding? Perhaps Columbine is giving you a reminder to appreciate, nurture, and love yourself and all the goodness that life offers you. Columbine offers healing energy right where it is needed. This card reflects a wonderful treasure to capture the beauty of life and the beauty within, allowing you to feel and express your Divine beauty.

Energy Impact (chakra correspondence)
3rd and 7th chakras

Affirmations
"I treasure my inner gifts and willingly share these gifts with others."

"I capture the beauty of life, opening myself up to my own Divine beauty, within and without."

"I embrace myself in golden yellow light."

44

COMFREY

(Symphytum officinale)
PRIMARY QUALITY: SERVICE

Voice of the Flower
"I am a strong, wise, and vulnerable helper who is here to serve you unconditionally. Yet I need to take time for personal retreat. It is necessary that I protect myself to balance the energy that I give out. It may be difficult to get to know me, but once you find the doorway open, you will discover my capacity for endless compassion. It is through my compassion that I am so very drawn to offer my service to you. I offer you the gift of compassion and greater

understanding in rising above the mundane and seeing the greater good of your situation. By so doing, you will be able to freely give of yourself and to offer your services when needed. Service is a gift that comes from the heart, free of conditions, free of entanglements."

Insight

When you choose the Comfrey card, there may be a calling from somewhere deep inside of you that is reaching toward a spiritual vision, an inner wisdom that is aware that a personal sacrifice may be needed in order to serve the highest good of all concerned. Comfrey teaches you to put things in perspective while staying connected to and in harmony with the whole. Comfrey offers protection and compassion, building a bridge between internal and external conditions while providing nurturing and solitude, prayer and meditation. Comfrey is giving you an opportunity to speak your truths from a place of spiritual knowing that comes from deep within, and to express harmony and balance in times when you are called to serve.

Energy Impact *(chakra correspondence)*
3rd, 4th, 5th, 6th, and 7th chakras

Affirmations

"I seek spiritual guidance and pray for truth and awareness that will help me know the highest good of my circumstance."

"I am developing the capacity to help myself so that I can help others."

"I acknowledge that this is a cycle in my life in which personal service is needed. I will continue to be loved, protected, and nurtured while becoming an open vessel in serving the highest good of myself and humanity."

CRIMSON MONKEYFLOWER

(Mimulus cardinalis)

PRIMARY QUALITY: PERSONAL POWER

Voice of the Flower

"You will realize in me a doorway beyond personal limitation. Recognize in me that the doorway to your personal power is opened through your awareness and connection with the Divine power within you. As you focus on my qualities and drink the nectar of my free expression, you can resolve old patterns such as anger, fear, and shame that have been a burden to you and have harmed you. I am the doorway where each day you find a new opportunity to speak your truths, to heal the old, to invite the new. Come inside my red funnel and find the nectar deep within. My doorway awaits you. I call out to you to gather your strength. Claim your personal power and personal fulfillment."

Insight

When you choose the Crimson Monkeyflower card, you are being called to step into your personal power. Crimson Monkeyflower helps you to let go of sticky relationships or situations that you may find yourself in. It takes you back to your roots or past to heal any emotional bitterness and powerlessness that you may feel, helping you to tap into your own sweet nectar to gain or regain personal power by exploring, identifying, releasing, and working with your core emotions. Get in touch with how you have felt emotionally over the past month or so. What deep emotions are you holding onto? Where did they come from? How did they begin? Let yourself experience them. Breathe into the experience. Let yourself experience the creative power of this plant.

Energy Impact (chakra correspondence)

1st, 2nd, and 5th chakras

"I express my feelings from my place of highest good."

"I let go of relationships and circumstances that no longer serve me."

"The Divine in me is an infinite resource of personal power."

"I swim freely in a sea of emotions, continuously moving and flowing."

DESERT LARKSPUR

(Delphinium scaposum)

PRIMARY QUALITY: GRACEFUL PASSAGE

Voice of the Flower

"I am the sacred breath of the One who lives and breathes through you. Let my breath carry you deep inside my blue chamber. Hear my voice and song. My message is of change and movement. Whatever changes and growth you are resisting, it is now time to embrace those changes. Be as One with me, and breathe deep into the mystery of life. Use the power of your imagination and the clarity of your thoughts to transmute whatever it is that is holding you back. Take freedom in your flight and move with gracefulness as you ease into your life passages."

47

Insight

When you choose the Desert Larkspur card, you are given the gift of graceful passage. Desert Larkspur ignites a spark of inspiration that stirs excitement within and taps into your personal gifts, awakening your potential to embrace opportunities and to dance with life. Desert Larkspur enhances the power of your imagination and clarifies your thoughts and voice to transmit that which serves your highest good. You are entering a time of initiation and transformation. Take advantage of this moment. Allow the grace of Divine play to integrate into your work, play, and communication with others. Be willing to let go of the past and embrace the currents of energy you are now receiving. Your life is an adventure without limitations. Embrace it fully and gracefully.

Energy Impact (chakra correspondence)
5th and 6th chakras

Affirmations
"Change is a natural law of the universe. I embrace change gracefully as I ease into a new life passage."

"Light shines all the way through me and all around me as I take flight in my journey."

"I communicate easily and gracefully, listening to my breath, rhythm, tone, pattern, and sound."

"I express myself with grace and ease in every situation, and for the highest good of self and others."

DESERT MARIGOLD

(Baileya multiradiata)
PRIMARY QUALITY: FLEXIBILITY

Voice of the Flower
"Let my bright yellow color fill your mind and body with my warming presence. From my center, I pass on to you the wisdom that comes from deep within your soul. Trust this wisdom, and let your thoughts, emotions, and actions flow in your life circumstances. Honor your flexibility to move with any challenges or choices facing you in your daily life. May your heart and mind be filled with my yellow halo from deep within yourself, and may you feel the ability to be receptive and bend in even the slightest breeze."

Insight
When you choose this card, it may come at a time when more flexibility in your life is needed. Ask yourself if there is something you are overly attached to. Do you have a desire to understand how to deal with your attachment? In

what ways are you rigid? In what ways are you unwilling to negotiate? Is there something that you know you are overly attached to yet you don't know how to deal with the attachment?

Desert Marigold heightens your awareness and reminds you to silence your mind and become aware of your body and your present environment. From this place of heightened perception, allow yourself to be more accepting, flexible, and willing to flow with life's circumstances. Desert Marigold is here to teach you to balance your analytical mind with your intuition. Within this balance resides a fountain of wisdom. Let this wisdom guide you to nurture yourself and to find softness and flexibility in your own presence.

Energy Impact (chakra correspondence)
3rd chakra

Affirmations
"I honor my ability to be flexible and to flow with the challenges presented to me in my daily life."

"I trust the wisdom that comes from deep within, and I act according to the wisdom as I intuit and understand it."

"I give thanks for all that is given to me, and I bless the power of silence in my mind."

DESERT WILLOW

(Chilopsis linearis)

PRIMARY QUALITY: THE EMPRESS/COMPASSION

Voice of the Flower
"Oh children of the earth, hear my call. Come with me into the depths of my mystery and fill yourself with the nourishment of abundance and love. Search deeply inside and allow your heritage as a Divine child to be awakened. Listen

49

to my songs as you gently dance with the flow of your life's journey, expressing your inner Divine presence into the world. Your freedom will be restored as you open your heart toward the outpouring of love and compassion for all beings on this earth. As you give, so shall you receive.

"Remember to bless the children with the abundance of joy and love."

Insight

Desert Willow is a teacher of manifestation from within to without, allowing you to connect with your innermost sensations, thoughts, words, and feelings and manifest them into the world. When is the last time you took a candlelight bath, sat under a tree, or took time to do something special for yourself? Desert Willow beckons you to love, nurture, and nourish yourself. Take time to be with yourself in a way that fills you deep inside. When you choose the Desert Willow card, you are asked to search deep within to discover new ways to nurture, love, and give to yourself. Experience the authentic beauty of this flower and let your heart open to the compassion and love it gives to you. As you become familiar with this new sense of self, you are invited to share your compassion toward others, including the suffering of all humanity and earth life. The love that you give to others will be returned to you.

Energy Impact (chakra correspondence)
1st, 3rd, 4th, 5th, and 7th chakras

Affirmations
"I am loved and nourished every moment of every day."

"Honoring my ancient sensual nature, I allow myself to freely express it."

"I fertilize my thoughts and feelings with an abundant flow of compassion and beauty."

50

ECHINACEA

(Echinacea angustifolia)

PRIMARY QUALITY: REJUVENATION

Voice of the Flower

"I offer you my vitality for whatever it is that holds you back, that keeps you from renewing your energy and strength. I am here to help you eliminate old emotional patterns, thoughts, and actions, and all beliefs of sickness that exist in your memory of self, restoring you to wellness. The wind carries my seed and yours to foster a new place of growth, a refreshing place of becoming and being. Take this opportunity to renew and rejuvenate yourself, replacing the old with the inherent capacity for the new."

Insight

Fostering radiant health and vitality can restore your body-mind-soul to your natural, vibrant self. What your body really wants from you is to slow down and take care of it, to find ways that energize and revitalize your whole being. Sit quietly and ask yourself what you are feeling in the moment. Is there something that stands out to you? Is there a thought, feeling, or situation that lifts you up, holds you back, or brings you down? Getting in touch with what that is, notice how it affects your energy and wellness. Take some long and deep breaths, consciously releasing whatever it is that holds you back. Do things that give you life. Replace old eating habits with whole and fresh foods that feed your soul. Give your brain a break by getting out into nature and restoring your connection to yourself and to nature's bounty. Take time to move your body and breathe in fresh air, lifting your spirits. By creating a natural and healthy way to live, you will feel like a new person, energized and rejuvenated.

Energy Impact (chakra correspondence)
1st, 2nd, and 6th chakras

51

Affirmations

"I am the power of rejuvenation, of change, and of new growth."

"I am eliminating that which holds me back, and I am moving forward."

"I find deep satisfaction in letting go of the old and bringing in the new."

EVENING PRIMROSE

(Oenothera caespitosa)

PRIMARY QUALITY: INNER STRENGTH

Voice of the Flower

"My white light shines in the darkness of the night, giving full strength to my night blossoms and connecting me to the reflective light of La Luna, the Moon. I am comforted by her soft glowing strength and soothed by the brightness of her light. As a way shower, her Divine Mother moonlight is mirrored back to me, reminding me of my own feminine strength and inner reflections. It is here in the silence of the night that I sink my roots deep into the earth to find, gather, nurture, and cleanse all the parts of my being. Trusting my inner strength and the purity within, it is here that I find value and meaning in my relationship with self and all of life."

Insight

When you choose the Evening Primrose card, you are on a pathway of healing any unresolved issues centered around the heart. The Evening Primrose flower will help you to uncover any hidden emotional wounds, particularly related to your mother and, whether you are a man or woman, with your connection with your own feminine nature. Reflect upon your relationship with your mother, or a mother figure, and bring to your awareness how this relationship has influenced your inner strength and your relationship to your feminine self. If there has been an absence of a mother figure in your life,

52

allow yourself to get in touch with the feelings you have about this. Observe your feelings and thoughts. Evening Primrose is offering you an opportunity to reevaluate and reconnect with what it is that you truly value and honor most in life. Although this flower appears delicate, it's stronger than it seems and can grow from dry, rocky ground. It offers an awakening within, helping you to find your inner strength.

Energy Impact (chakra correspondence)
4th and 7th chakras

Affirmations
"I am guided by the light to the doorway of my soul."
"I honor and embrace my mother and myself unconditionally."
"The stillness of the night feeds my soul with comfort and strength."

HONEYSUCKLE

(Lonicera japonica halliana)
PRIMARY QUALITY: HARMONY

Voice of the Flower
"Open your hands as if to receive the warmth of the sun's radiant rays, and imagine the soles of your feet sinking into cool moist earth. Let the flow of energy move from your hands all the way to your feet. Now let the energy flow back from your feet and be received through your hands. Feeling this connection between your hands and feet, fill your senses. In this place I invite you to feel the presence of being in the moment now. Put aside all thoughts and emotions, letting your body-mind harmonize naturally with itself. Through the experience of this union, you will feel whole. Your thoughts, communications, and actions with others will bring harmony to yourself and to your life."

Insight

When you choose the Honeysuckle card, perhaps you are having difficulty maintaining your individuality in a partnership or with others. Old fears or nostalgic memories of the past may inhibit you from enjoying the sweetness of life at the present. By being present in the moment and connected with your whole person, you will feel a sense of peace and harmony within. Trust and accept your individuality. Honeysuckle brings together opposites (with self or others) in mutual balance, integration, and harmony. Experience the wholeness that harmony brings to you, giving you hope for new possibilities, and happiness in your life.

Energy Impact (chakra correspondence)
3rd and 7th chakras

Affirmations
"I have the power to integrate all that I am and all that I am becoming."

"I am willing to reconcile with my opposites and bring harmony and balance from deep within."

"Allowing the flow of energy within my being, I bring peace and harmony to my thoughts and actions."

INDIAN PAINTBRUSH

(*Castilleja chromosa*)
PRIMARY QUALITY: CREATIVITY

Voice of the Flower

"I invite you to enter the silence of mind where no voice is heard and no sound is made. In this deep stillness you will feel my presence. Allow your roots, at the deepest core of your being, to draw upon my resources. You will come to realize that no matter where you came from or who you are, you have the ability to create within yourself a new sense of wholeness. Experience the silence in me, and in this place you will feel the fullness of survival in your world. You will discover a newfound freedom, allowing you to break through your dependencies with others and live a life of interdependence.

"My silence will inspire your vision, your passion for life, and your creativity for living. With each moment, you are creating your life."

Insight

The Indian Paintbrush card is a reminder to take time out from your daily life to be still and to relax in silence. Through silence, you can feel connected within. From this place of wholeness, in the midst of a silent mind and body, healing occurs. You will feel a stirring of creativity and inspiration. New insights and life visions may arrive at your doorstep. You may discover a newfound freedom of living a more interdependent life with others, increasing your awareness of any relationship in which one person is too dependent upon another or understanding the times in your life when you are dependent on others. Staying connected to your roots and resources, allow yourself to fully express your life passions. Let your inspirations guide you to live a fulfilling and creative life.

Energy Impact (chakra correspondence)
1st, 2nd, 4th, and 6th chakras

Affirmations
"I feel relaxed and rooted in who I am, knowing that my needs are met easily and creatively."

"In the stillness of mind and body, I feel the power of my presence."

"I love myself for who I am, and through love of myself, I creatively express compassion toward humanity and all earth life."

LUPINE

(Lupinus argentus)
PRIMARY QUALITY: PATHFINDER

Voice of the Flower
"I am a way shower, here to help you observe the way you receive and use your abilities, make choices, and discover your true path as you walk your life's journey. You will come to understand that the power within you is based on your capacity to know yourself. Receive my guidance, and let me illuminate you along your path. Feel the power of my presence enter and energize your body-mind-soul. In the stillness of this moment, allow that step to take place between what was and what will become. In this place, let light fill your silence and carry your vision. It will take you beyond time and space. This is the meaning of the Pathfinder."

Insight
When you get the Lupine card, you may be on a path of healing or a path to finding a higher purpose or deeper meaning to life. Lupine gives you the ability to step beyond yourself, helping you to attain your vision and to bring it into physical application. By doing so, you will enrich yourself and others and your life choices. Acknowledge the silence or space of being that Lupine offers you, and let yourself be in that space without looking ahead or behind. Feel a natural flow of energy take place. This is the experience of a Pathfinder.

Energy Impact (chakra correspondence)
6th and 7th chakras

Affirmations
"I open my hands to receive the power of light."
"My pathway is illuminated by my intuition and inner silence."
"I honor my evolutionary growth and surrender to my highest good."

MEXICAN HAT

(Ratibida columnaris)
PRIMARY QUALITY: RELEASE

Voice of the Flower

"Come sit under my flowering canopy and allow yourself to rest and release. May you feel protected under my canopy, and experience the freedom to express and reflect that which you feel bound by. Allow me to help you encounter that which lies beneath your pains and suffering. By meeting that which brings you pain and experiencing each pain for what it is, its power over you is released. Give yourself this opportunity to free up those places inside of you that need healing. Allow the earth to share your burdens, and feel her strength and support. Stand true to your own power as you experience release."

Insight

Mexican Hat helps you to look at that which gives you pain so you can let go of the pain and whatever it is that holds you back. As you face each pain and experience the pain for what it is, it can no longer have power over you. With each release, you will experience healing from deep within. By surrendering to your highest good, and releasing your burdens, Mexican Hat offers you a pathway of wholeness that gives you guidance and support, nourishing yourself, your environment, and the earth you live on.

Energy Impact (chakra correspondence)
1st, 2nd, and 3rd chakras

Affirmations
"I surrender my hold on pain and turn it over to God."
"I let go of (name a situation or a person) and pray for the highest good."
"May the burdens I am choosing to carry be released."

MORNING GLORY

(Ipomoea purpurea)

PRIMARY QUALITY: LIBERATOR

Voice of the Flower

"My splendor shines forth in exaltation and celebration of the dawning of a new day. As the sun begins its journey in the east, I, too, open up my petals and embrace the beginning of a new day. I offer you the awareness to begin anew. May you feel liberated for just one moment in my presence, completely free of worry and doubt. And may this moment guide and awaken you to ignite the spark of beginning a new life, of making a fresh start. Let your heart sing out in glorious praise as you embark upon your new journey. Receive the generosity and vitality of my nature. My invitation to you is to give yourself the permission to break away from old patterns, and embrace the light that is inherent within you. Let my essence help you begin a new step toward Self liberation."

Insight

58 Look at the Morning Glory card and notice the soft and gentle glow in the center of the flower. Breathe into the presence of this glow and let it enter your being. As you exhale, bring your awareness to the deep magenta star that reaches toward the edges of the flower and the violet-purple color of the petals. How do you feel when you look at Morning Glory? What do you see? Morning Glory helps you to be in touch with your natural rhythms, to overcome sluggishness, to sleep deeply, and to awake refreshed. Morning Glory offers a freeing or liberation of the Self that is guided by a Higher Power, stimulating vitality and your ability to make a fresh start. If you are seeking inspiration, compassion, and a new outlook toward life, Morning Glory is for you! Perhaps the beautiful glowing colors of the Morning Glory will beckon you to get up in the morning and to take the time to watch a sunrise.

Energy Impact (chakra correspondence)
4th, 6th, and 7th chakras

Affirmations
"May the love in my heart flow within me and outside of me to every living
thing."
"May the light within me shine forth and illuminate my path, keeping my
mind clear and aware in this moment now."
"I celebrate this day with a new thought, a new feeling, and a new activity."

MULLEIN
(Verbascum thapsus)
PRIMARY QUALITY: SECURITY

Voice of the Flower
"I have a powerful ability to take in and to absorb that which feeds my life,
my spirit, and my growth. I will show you the benefit of taking in and incor-
porating what it is that you have the ability to absorb at the highest level possible. As you awaken and stir your unconscious mind, you will learn to live
and act according to your inner truths and values. As my lemon-cupped flowers and seeds are securely shielded in my soft and woolly flesh, I offer you
security and protection. By trusting in your own inner resources and by not
looking outside yourself, you can experience a true sense of security. Here
you will learn to listen to your inner voice. Experience my intimate nature, my
gentle strength, and my soft touch."

Insight
When you get the Mullein card, you may be on a pathway of wholeness that
seeks intimacy and security within yourself as well as within all of your relationships. Mullein is especially helpful for men or women who want to strengthen

yet soften their masculine nature. Mullein promotes strength with gentleness, enhancing intimacy and humility. Mullein teaches you to listen to your inner voice and to live and act according to your inner truths and values.

Energy Impact (chakra correspondence)
2nd and 3rd chakras

Affirmations
"I give myself time each day to listen to and understand myself, appreciating my self-worth."

"I am guided by my inner light and am focused toward a positive direction in my life."

"I find intimacy, security, and gentleness within myself."

ONION

(Allium cepa)
PRIMARY QUALITY: MEMBERSHIP

Voice of the Flower
"I welcome you to explore beneath the surface of your being. I am here to help you discover the layers of consciousness beyond your illusion of fear and separation. During your journey, as each layer dissolves, you become more and more aware of your true nature. The layers of separation and fear peel away. You bring to your awareness, union and connection with every living thing. Your universal child is born, and you find your place in the world."

Insight
When you choose the Onion card, you may be coming to new terms with yourself. Perhaps you are being given an opportunity to peel away yet another layer within yourself, bringing to you peace and unity. By doing so, you may discover

a new depth of understanding about yourself and how you fit into the world around you. As you experience this connection with yourself and let go of that layer which has been suppressed, your heart and mind open. You have a deeper understanding about your relationship to your whole self, and you naturally come to terms with where you belong and how you become a member of that belonging.

Energy Impact (chakra correspondence)
4th and 7th chakras

Affirmations
"May the light within me fill my heart with peace."

"As I peel off my inner layers, I am discovering a newfound freedom of giving energy to myself and others."

"I am embodied by the One who lives and breathes through me, and I see all of the universe as an embodiment of one Source."

OX-EYE DAISY

(Chrysanthemum leucanthemum)
PRIMARY QUALITY: INNER KNOWING

Voice of the Flower
"Let my presence help you tap into your higher consciousness to expand your thoughts and emotions. From this place of expansion, you will learn to live life from a place of inner awareness. By acting in harmony with the natural rhythm from within, you will feel at peace with yourself, feeling supported by your decisions and thoughts. By connecting with and trusting your inner knowing, you will discover the balance between this and your intelligence, for both carry each other. Honor the wisdom from within your mind's eye, and let that wisdom support and nurture what it is that you feel inside. Let yourself enjoy happiness. Come laugh, sing, and play with me."

Insight
When you choose the Ox-Eye Daisy card, you are asked to listen to what you feel and know from within to help you in the decisions that you make. When you make decisions only from your intellect, you may overlook or mistrust your inner voice. Although your decision may appear rational, it may not be made for your highest good. Ox-Eye Daisy teaches you the balance between intellect and intuition. By integrating your inner knowing with your intellect, you will gain wisdom, understanding, vision, and clarity as you make choices along your life's path. If you are in need of living a more optimistic, fun-loving life, Ox-Eye Daisy is a good flower for you. It reminds us to live life more fully, to enjoy children, and to bring play and laughter into our everyday routines.

Energy Impact (chakra correspondence)
3rd and 7th chakras

Affirmations
"My thoughts are a reflection of who I am. The higher my thoughts, the freer I feel."

"May I walk in harmony with the natural rhythm I feel from within."

"I honor and trust my inner knowing when I make decisions and life choices."

PALMER'S PENSTEMON

(Penstemon palmeri)
PRIMARY QUALITY: SELF-EXPRESSION

Voice of the Flower
"To speak from the heart is the gift I offer you. Inside my soft pink chambers you will find my inner essence filled with the sweet taste of nectar and

compassion. Take in my nectar and allow it to fill your heart, mind, and soul. Feel the warmth of compassion and imagine my soft pink glow within your heart and all around it. Bring this glow and the compassion you feel with you as you step outside the chamber and into the opening of my petals. Become aware of any sounds you make and how you make them. Listen to the words you say and how you say them. Express yourself from the heart, and notice how the world around you responds."

Insight
When you choose the Palmer's Penstemon card, you are being asked to look carefully at the ways in which you express yourself. Perhaps you are suppressed in some way that you communicate or you may speak from reactions of the mind or emotions. Palmer's Penstemon inspires you to experiment with new patterns of speech and communication in a heartfelt and honest way that voices your true feelings and thoughts. By doing so, you will feel your heart open and soon discover that others may respond to you with a greater depth of sensitivity, valuing what you say and how you say it. Perhaps you will also notice your capacity for being a better listener.

63

Energy Impact (chakra correspondence)
3rd, 4th, 5th, and 6th chakras

Affirmations
"I embrace the highest good of all when I speak my truths."

"I am mindful of my bitterness, and I create a new and positive pattern of self-expression."

"I allow the air of my body to communicate from deep within my heart."

PALOVERDE

(Cercidium floridum)
PRIMARY QUALITY: EARTH WISDOM

Voice of the Flower

"It is my soil, my sacred ground, that I bring to your awareness, your own inner sanctuary. By connecting within, you become more aligned with universal earth laws as opposed to man-made laws. This allows you to tap into your wisdom, the wisdom that is already inherent within you. Authentic wisdom is not based on outside conditions or what others tell you, but it is a wisdom that comes from within. As you go through life planting seeds of wisdom in your choices and in your relations, you will soon discover the value of making wiser choices in your life. You will take into consideration the larger whole. Sometimes one's decisions may draw unwanted consequences, yet based on a deeper connection within your self, you may experience the inherent wisdom of a lesson learned. If you truly made a connection, the outcome would be based more on self-authenticity and aligned with who you are. As you walk in harmony on the earth, you are reenacting your role as a cocreator to sustain earth life. This is the foundation of grace in the world and the wisdom from which it survives."

Insight

When you choose the Paloverde card, you may be on a pathway of healing that yearns to connect and relate to the earth as a provider and resource, not only in the physical form but in all forms. The Paloverde flower helps you to ground and connect with the wisdom and gifts that the earth provides, which are inherent within you. By aligning yourself with universal values such as ecological and environmental awareness, quality of life for all, and lifestyle consciousness, you are tapping into your natural wisdom. You begin to take into consideration the larger whole, aware of the consequences of the decisions you make. You find that you become more aligned to who you are, and your experiences and life choices become authentic to your nature.

You are given an opportunity to walk in harmony on the earth and to find ways to sustain her, yourself, your family, and all your relations.

Energy Impact (chakra correspondence)
1st, 2nd, and 3rd chakras

Affirmations
"Mother, carry me in the wisdom of your deep blue sea
 Mother, hold me in the wisdom of humility.
 Mother, carry me in the wisdom of your deep rich earth
 Mother, hold me in the wisdom of my new birth."

"I see the higher truth in all things, and I exist as an equal to all of life."

"I allow the earth of my body to nurture me."

PEACE ROSE

(Rosa peace)

PRIMARY QUALITY: GIFT OF THE ANGELS

Voice of the Flower
"Within all the thorns that are presented in your life, your pains, sufferings, challenges, and even your hard work, my gentle and endearing presence is always here. When you have lost all hope and feel out of touch with love, I will help you gather your courage and find the faith to go deeper inside your pain. You will discover that even within the deepest pain, there is the gift of peace and love. My flower, like an angel, gives you the gifts of beauty, love, courage, and peace. Be as One with me. Allow yourself to emerge as a flower, inspired by love, and set your heart free."

Insight

When you choose the Peace Rose card, you may feel your heart is closed, or you might be feeling shut down in some way. Perhaps you are suffering from depression or grieving the loss of a loved one. It is time to no longer be held back by life's thorns. Nothing remains the same nor is it like it was. There is always a bigger picture that God has planned to help us grow, love, and let go, and to help us grieve in our sorrow, feeling the pain, so that we can again become the flower. The flowers bloom according to the season. We, too, bloom in relation to our life cycles. Sometimes there are only a few blossoms on one rose bush, and other times, there are many more. The Peace Rose flower gives you the courage and faith to face your pains and suffering, inspiring you to accept life's cycles and to open your heart to receive love, joy, peace, and beauty. Perhaps Peace Rose is giving you an opportunity to help you to come to terms with what it is that you value within yourself. By loving yourself, you will have more love to share with others.

Energy Impact (chakra correspondence)
1st, 4th, and 7th chakras

66

Affirmations
"I honor the beauty of all of life and all of life's passings."

"My pains and sufferings are inspired by my hope and love."

"My heart is a vessel of love, my mind is a vessel of truth. My body is a vessel of healing."

PINYON

(Pinus edulis)

PRIMARY QUALITY: ENDURING PATIENCE

Voice of the Flower

"I am a teacher of great patience and perseverance, honoring the process of steady growth and slow maturation. I offer you patience for your personal growth without shame, guilt, or time restraints. Accept who you are and take on a new effort to further explore and develop a new sense of self. Develop your foundation. Be strong and enduring. Come to terms with yourself and make dependable choices. As you let go of past errors and mistakes, you will feel less burdened. A newfound freedom will be felt, and you will bear the fruits of your enduring patience."

Insight

This may be an opportunity for you to take time for yourself, to let go of your shortcomings, and to allow what is to be. The conelets on the Pinyon tree take twenty-six months to evolve and are a reflection of the Pinyon's patience and perseverance. The slow but steady maturation of the tree and its pine nuts can also teach you to be patient and persevering in your own life so that you, too, can bear your fruits through your steadfast endurance. Breathe in the scent of the Pinyon's resin and pine needles; its refreshing presence will invite you in.

67

Energy Impact (chakra correspondence)

1st, 4th, and 6th chakras

Affirmations

"I am free to love myself and others without shame, blame, or guilt."

"I live patiently in the moment thanking my Creator for all that I am."

"I allow the body of the earth to nurture my roots."

POMEGRANATE

(Punica granatum)
PRIMARY QUALITY: FRUIT OF LIFE

Voice of the Flower

"Come with me into my flaming orange petals and embrace the darkness where your innate wisdom lies. Allow me to stir your deepest passions, joys, and creativity, awakening your vital life force energy. Celebrate the fullness of your sensuality. Here in the darkness, discover your primal feminine self uniting with the Divine Earth Mother. Receive the fruits of her abundance and beauty, and honor them within yourself. Drawing upon your resources, treasure these gifts as you delight in your freedom, expressing your passion for life and for living."

Insight

When you choose the Pomegranate card, perhaps you are struggling in some way to find enough abundance to support yourself in the world. Pomegranate attracts an abundance of positive, fruitful inner and outer resources, guiding you toward personal balance within yourself, at home, with your family, and in your role in the larger community. Pomegranate stirs passion, creative awareness, and expression of feminine energy, nurturing you and connecting you with Nature. Pomegranate is a teacher of your inner wisdom, beauty, and power in the seemingly darkest moments of your life. By setting healthy boundaries, you will learn to express your emotions and creativity in safe ways, feeling free in who you are.

Energy Impact (chakra correspondence)
1st, 2nd, and 3rd chakras

Affirmations

"I flow infinitely and passionately from within, greeting life with joyful abundance."

"My power is filled with the fruits of my deepest creativity."

"I nurture my emotions and embrace my creative nature, from which I attract an abundant flow of resources."

PURPLE ROBE

(Nierembergia)

PRIMARY QUALITY: PLENTY

Voice of the Flower

"My message to you is to show you that you cannot be limited and that supply is the law of expansion and fruition. The universe supplies us with infinite resources, from within ourselves to outside of ourselves. The creative feminine principle of creation and reproduction is a continual process of harvesting the fruits of your thoughts and actions as you fill your heart, mind, body, and soul with goodness from within and goodness for all. She overflows in limitless, boundless, and abundant energy, and she offers to you a splendor of excess in every breath you take. Take in my spirit of plenty and fill yourself with boundless treasures."

Insight

When you choose the Purple Robe card, perhaps you are on a pathway of healing where the feeling of lack in your life is replaced with the feeling of plenty. Purple Robe is prolific, widely spread, producing an abundance of flowers. It demonstrates its quality of plenty by the way it grows and produces. The cupped flowers appear delicate although the petals are actually quite strong and pronounced. These signatures give a sense of strength and

69

persistence to grow and spread, offering a gentle approach in doing so. The rich purple color of the flower is characteristic of the brow energy center, giving you a sense of purpose, spiritual insight, and wisdom. Experience the abundance of the Purple Robe, and deepen your awareness and vision of the supply already inherent within you.

Energy Impact (chakra correspondence)
3rd and 6th chakras

Affirmations
"There is an unlimited supply in my life. I have the choice to create it."

"I am limitless, boundless, and filled with abundant energy."

"I creatively weave my thoughts, my visions, my imaginations, and my inspirations to manifest that which will abundantly serve my highest good."

SAGE

(Salvia Officinalis-purpurascens)
PRIMARY QUALITY: WHOLE-LIFE INTEGRATION

Voice of the Flower
"Step inside my cool chambers and hear my sacred voice. I offer you guidance on a path toward wholeness by helping you to become consciously aware of how you integrate your higher purpose in life with your daily life patterns of living. Your presence in the world is shown to yourself and others in the ways that you act, live, think, express, and relate. By merging your spiritual intention with the way you live your life, you will feel whole and connected. Listen to my sounds, take in my refreshing breath, and experience a cleansing of your body, soul, and mind. I invite you to come fully into your Divine presence with your own voice and song through sounds, speech, touch, and senses. May you feel whole through this connection with yourself, allowing the feeling of wholeness to bring integration into your life."

Insight

When you choose the Sage card, you may become more aware of the sounds you make and the words that you choose to communicate with others. You may come to an understanding with yourself in the ways that you integrate your spirituality with practical applications of daily living and how you behave in the world. Sage offers spiritual inspiration and visionary guidance and is useful in times of transition and life-cycle changes. Hear the Sage beckon you toward higher life purposes and more conscious ways of living and being, bringing wholeness within and without.

Energy Impact (chakra correspondence)

1st, 3rd, 4th, 5th, and 7th chakras

Affirmations

"I open my inner doorway and step inside the core of my being."

"My voice is a vessel of sound, speaking my truth all around."

"I allow the Light of my body to guide and fill me."

SAGUARO

(Cereus Giganteus)

PRIMARY QUALITY: THE GUARDIAN

Voice of the Flower

"Help me build a strong nation of people who stand by their truths, who guard against ill ways of being and living, who protect their children and their environment, and who live with dignity. I will show you how to endure and how to live with great strength, insight, wisdom, and humbleness. Through my connection with the ancestors, I will help you gain access to the resources and reserves from deep within yourself and outside of yourself. Enter the stillness of my presence, and honor all that is sacred. Take time out every day for prayer, silence, and devotion."

Insight
When you choose the Saguaro card, you may be learning how to persevere in times of struggle and how to build up your own reserves in times of need. The Saguaro helps you to feel rooted and balanced, awakening and stimulating each sacred energy center, from the root to the crown. It offers cleansing and releases stagnation and tension at all levels throughout the body, helping you to restore, stretch, and expand beyond any self-imposed limitations. You may experience your consciousness expanding as you get a sense of a deeper purpose in your life and embrace new ways of thought, actions, and choices. Saguaro, the guardian ancestor of the desert, teaches you to protect yourself, your children, and your environment, to live with honor and in truth. Experience the power of this desert giant, and feel its presence within you.

Energy Impact (chakra correspondence)
1st, 4th, and 7th chakras

72

Affirmations
"I release and expand at all levels of my being, inviting the Divine to guide my thoughts and actions."

"I protect, honor, and respect all that is sacred and that all are sacred."

"I am patient and enduring, strong yet humble."

SCARLET PENSTEMON

(Penstemon barbatus)
PRIMARY QUALITY: COURAGE

Voice of the Flower
"My message to you is to accept life's painful challenges as lessons to rebuild your faith and to have the courage and strength to take the next step forward. Seek your inner guidance and find the inner strength to go deep inside yourself. Take a sip of your sweet nectar and feel the courage to be vulnerable to love and to be loving. Find the courage to be soft and nurturing, the courage to share your passion with your lover. It takes courage and the willingness to take risks in order to follow your higher life's path. And it takes even more courage to face life's setbacks and to trust that you are being provided for."

Insight
When you choose the Scarlet Penstemon card, you may in some way lack the courage and confidence needed to draw positive change to your life. Scarlet Penstemon offers you strength and vitality to face life's challenges, to rebuild your faith, and to stand on your own two feet. The flower faces downward as an expression of surrender. Its long, narrow tube contains sweet nectar deep inside. Imagine the strength and courage needed to go deep within yourself, finding your nectar, the essence of your being. Once the nectar is found, its sweet taste comforts and nurtures you. It gives you the courage to be yourself in the way you feel, think, and act and to have the courage to be vulnerable to love and to be loving.

Energy Impact (chakra correspondence)
1st, 2nd, 3rd, and 5th chakras

73

Affirmations

"God grant me the serenity to accept the things I cannot change, the courage to change the things I can, and the wisdom to know the difference."—The Serenity Prayer

"I have the courage to let go of the old and the courage to bring in the new."

"I have the courage to go deep inside myself, to be vulnerable to love and to be loving."

STRAWBERRY HEDGEHOG

(Echinocereus engelmannii)
PRIMARY QUALITY: PASSION

Voice of the Flower

"I have great passion for living, for appreciating and loving the pleasures life has to offer me. The secret of enjoying these magnificent pleasures is to open your heart and tap into your ecstatic nature. The desire realms within your heart will open your passion for joy and pleasure. I awaken within you the sacred energy that rises up the spine, spiraling to the heart and out the top of the head. Celebrate the union of this ecstatic energy and take in its presence. Enjoy life as a celebration of discovery and spontaneous activity. Allow yourself to be in the moment now and avoid thinking about what you didn't do yesterday and what you need to do next. Become so absorbed by my spirit of passion and the fullness of the moment that nothing else matters now. Give yourself permission to be completely and unconditionally receptive to the celebration of your own creative passion and pleasures."

Insight

Reflect upon the ways that you block passion in your life. Notice your thoughts and feelings and any body awareness in your response to this reflection. Now reflect upon the ways that you are passionate, creative, and celebrate life.

Notice how you feel when you connect with your passion. The miraculous power of this beautiful, sensual flower has the capacity to emerge through a cluster of spines that surrounds and protects it. With a burst of passion, the Strawberry Hedgehog flower embodies freedom that blooms in spite of difficult circumstances. The passionate magenta petals of the flower are strong, yet yielding and gentle. Strawberry Hedgehog cultivates relationships and sensual openness based on trust, security, protection, intimacy, and expressing love freely and passionately. Enjoy the passion of this flower as you open yourself up to love and compassion. Your pathway of healing is about appreciating yourself and all that is good in your life. Take this moment to celebrate life! Perhaps you will be inspired to dance, sing, write, create, or celebrate life with passion and love.

Energy Impact (chakra correspondence)
1st, 3rd, and 4th chakras

Affirmations
"I am an abundant resource, giving love and receiving love."

"I allow the creative sensual petals of my personality to burst forth and to receive, give, and share in life's celebration."

"I unconditionally allow myself to passionately receive and express the pleasures of blissful love."

SUNFLOWER

(Helianthus Annuus)
PRIMARY QUALITY: FOUNTAIN OF YOUTH

Voice of the Flower
"As the sun rises in the east, I awake refreshed as my flower head faces the sun to meet a new day. In the center of my flower's disk, I feel an opening, an

expansion, from the warmth and light of the sun. Slowly my petals stretch further outward. Moment by moment, throughout the day, I turn toward the sun, basking in its rays, I let its light into me. Turn toward me and follow the light. I will unite you with the source of love and power and help you find your deepest sense of purpose that you came into this life with. Only you know what your life purpose is and how you will manifest it. Feel the light enter the soles of your feet and let it move up your legs to your belly. Feel warmth from deep within you and all around you. Allow wisdom and strength to embellish you, to take you in, and to hold you in that place. Here you will feel an incredible sense of purpose and power. Let your sun shine. Trust in yourself. Bring the child alive that is within you!"

Insight
When you choose the Sunflower card, you are being guided by the power of the sun, letting its radiant light shine on you wherever you turn. Bring your awareness to those aspects in yourself that give you joy, optimism, and a feeling of purpose and power. Notice your thoughts and feelings and your physical body. Sunflower restores youth and innocence, fun and play, liveliness and pleasure, bringing life to the child within you and directing you toward purpose and positive thought, joy, and humor. The sun is known to represent the male energy within you, giving you the ability to assert yourself in the world with positive determination, optimism, and direction. Sunflower gives you the ability to think and reason, to gather strength and power from deep within. Feel the warmth of the sun shine down upon you, and give thanks for its expansive energy.

Energy Impact (chakra correspondence)
3rd chakra

Affirmations
"I am renewed by my purpose in life, finding ways to bring it to manifestation."

"I allow my personal power to shine from deep within my roots and outward toward the sun."

"I am empowered to create loving thoughts and circumstances from a place of joy, wisdom, and strength."

SWEET PEA

(Lathyrus latifolius)
PRIMARY QUALITY: GROWING CHILD

Voice of the Flower

"Within my tender folds, I offer you a place of security and protection. In this place, you will feel my great compassion and taste my sweet essence. I give you the strength to love yourself unconditionally and to nurture yourself as you change and grow. Prevent yourself from trying to make everything happen so fast in your life. Honor yourself and embrace your personal growth as you walk your journey. Slow down and pace yourself. By doing so, you will experience the freedom to be your authentic, natural self. You will have the ability to radiate your personal power and creative loving energy with your family members, friends, and the world at large."

Insight

When you choose the Sweet Pea card, notice the broad, hood-shaped petal that looks as if a child is sitting with a hood or cap over its head. Inside the hood, the child feels safe, calm, and secure. The two smaller side petals that resemble wings indicate freedom, and the two folding lower petals also offer the flower's character of protection and security. The climbing feature of the Sweet Pea, whereby the vines need a support structure to grow on, represents the child's gradual growth process and the support needed to find secure footholds by which to gain confidence and emotional security as the child enters the larger world. Sweet Pea has a soft, gentle beauty which opens the heart, teaching you to love yourself and others unconditionally. It's a reminder of the gentleness and compassion needed to raise a child and to love the authentic child within.

Energy Impact (chakra correspondence)
4th chakra

Affirmations
"I appreciate and love who I am, acknowledging my pleasures and my pains."

"I have the capacity to appreciate being alone yet knowing when to integrate and participate in the world around me."

"I make choices in my life that feed my personal growth and give me a strong sense of security."

THISTLE

(Circium neomexicanum)
PRIMARY QUALITY: BALANCE

Voice of the Flower
"It is the center of my sacred circle that holds the power of union between inner and outer, hard and soft, light and dark, sweet and bitter. It is at this center where the balance of Divine presence, vision, light, wisdom, and communication from above meet with matter, survival, procreation, knowledge, and personality from below. When your heart is open, a natural balance of energy and power radiates from your center. The center allows light to enter within and darkness to reach its void. It allows the magic within you to feel a deep sense of peace and contentment."

Insight
When you choose the Thistle card, you may be on a pathway of healing that is searching for balance in your life. Bring your awareness to any parts of your-

self or to situations that prevent you from connecting with your true self. Identify those parts as best as you can and observe your response to this awareness. Now take some time to reflect upon experiences that have given you a sense of being centered, whole, and in balance with yourself. Thistle assists you in softening your character if needed or in protecting yourself in those circumstances where you need to bear those thorny edges. You may experience that place within yourself where the darkness meets the light, giving you a feeling of being centered and in balance. This allows your heart center to open and radiate a creative force of energy and power. Feel this energy within and around your heart, circling outward. Take in the special presence of this flower, and experience your wholeness.

Energy Impact (chakra correspondence)
4th, 6th, and 7th chakras

Affirmations
"Darkness will ultimately be lost in the light of transforming love."
"As I breathe deep into my heart, I feel balanced and centered."
"I allow any rough edges of my personality to feel soft from deep within."
"I take time to be with myself, finding my center."

VERVAIN

(Verbena macdougali)

PRIMARY QUALITY: REACH FOR THE STARS

Voice of the Flower
"As each circle of flowers moves upward along my stem, I remain open to the journey of every moment as it reveals itself to me. As my roots sink deeper into the earth and my spiral grows higher toward the sky, I feel hope and joy inside that I am on a path of higher direction. Releasing any tensions along the

way, my personal growth unfolds. Inspired to hold my vision and to enjoy my journey, moment by moment, I reach for my destiny. May you experience my light shining forth like brilliant stars lighting your way."

Insight
When you choose the Vervain card, perhaps you are on a path of healing that brings simplicity and moderation without complication or extreme measures. Ask yourself the following questions. What can I do to help myself achieve a long awaited goal? How can I achieve this goal while staying down to earth and taking responsibility for my daily life activities? How can I simplify my life while striving for and staying focused on my goals? Vervain gives you the insight and perspective to see what lies ahead, allowing you to remain relaxed, grounded, and focused while you carry out each step along the way. By doing so, the direction and leadership you take will influence your life choices and will give you a sense of crowning achievement. Stay open and tolerant with others, helping them on their own path of healing.

Energy Impact (chakra correspondence)

6th and 7th chakras

Affirmations
"I value each step along my path as I get closer to my vision and my life goals."

"My commitment to myself today is to engage in an activity that releases stress and tension."

"I make conscious thoughts and actions that give me inspiration and hope."

WILD ROSE

(Rosa arizonaca)
PRIMARY QUALITY: LOVE

Voice of the Flower
"I invite you to open your heart and receive the love that is already inherent within you. May you find an opening within your heart to love the gift of being alive. Embrace each opportunity to face your challenges and your pains and to find release from your miseries. Letting go of your resistance to loving life, you will have the capacity to love yourself. By giving yourself to love, you are investing in nourishing your heart with a continual flow of blood and circulation throughout your body filled with harmonious and loving thoughts and feelings. I am the love within you singing deep into your heart."

Insight
When you choose Wild Rose, you are drawing to yourself the power of love, compassion, and joy for living. The Wild Rose card is calling you to discover the love already inherent within you and to live your life by listening to your heart. Only you have the ability to make your own life choices according to what you love in your life. You may begin to notice more clearly how your emotions and thoughts influence the way you love and are loved. If you are grieving the loss of a loved one, feeling a lack of love in your life, indifferent, unmotivated, or feeling despair in any way, may you open the doorway in your heart for the power of love to pour through you. Give yourself to love and nourish your heart, mind, body, and soul.

Energy Impact (chakra correspondence)
3rd and 4th chakras

Affirmations

"I give myself to love, nourishing my heart, body, mind, and soul."

"I release my deepest heartaches and devote myself to love."

"I begin this day in love and live in love all day long."

WILLOW

(Salix Gooddingii)

PRIMARY QUALITY: FORGIVENESS

Voice of the Flower

"I protect the flowing waters that live beside me. I am nurtured by the waters as my roots sink deep into the earth. I am trustworthy and flexible, and my hearty branches bend and sway gracefully in the wind. If you try to force me, my branch will snap, causing me to break down. My taste becomes bitter. You will, however, feel my strength and endurance in your ability and desire to forgive under any circumstances and to release any sadness or resentment you may feel. You will get to know me by my generosity and by my willingness to stretch and bend."

82

Insight

When you choose the Willow card, you may be coming to an understanding of the root cause of any resentment, bitterness, or even sadness that you are holding onto. Perhaps you are now willing to forgive yourself or others, or at least more willing to look at what it is you need to forgive. Reflecting upon yourself, you may want to ask yourself in what ways you hold resentment, bitterness, or sadness. Is there someone in your life whom you need to forgive? Is there something in yourself that needs forgiveness? Observe your thoughts and feelings and any body awareness that comes to you as you contemplate these questions. Now take some time to look at the way you provide structure in your life and how you move with the ebb and flow of change. You may ask yourself "In what ways am I rigid, going against the flow in my life?" Again, notice your thoughts and feelings. Willow teaches you to be flexible in your approach to life and all living things and to move with the ebb and flow of life's wisdom and grace. Let the grace of Willow open your heart and present an opportunity in your life to share an act of forgiving kindness toward another.

Energy Impact (chakra correspondence)
4th and 7th chakras

Affirmations
"I bend gracefully with opportunities that are presented to me."

"I allow the waters of life to flow and weave throughout my body-mind-soul bestowing agility, flexibility, and a deep level of forgiveness."

"As I am generous and forgiving of myself and others, all resentments are released."

YARROW

(Achillea Millefolium)
PRIMARY QUALITY: PROTECTION

Voice of the Flower
"My soft, delicate leaves appear feathery and light. Yet the potency of their healing qualities behold a shield of protection within you and all around you. May you capture the glow of my bone-white petals, feeling energized and protected by their warmth.

"Allow yourself to live life and make choices that give you security from within to without. When you feel your energy is depleted by others, by life circumstances, or even by yourself, you can make the choice to guard against unwanted influences. Creating security within yourself, feeling safe and free, you have the choice to protect the ways in which you extend your energy. Experience the power of my nurturing presence, and relieve yourself of any tensions. Protecting the energy you give out, you allow healing to take place."

Insight

When you choose the Yarrow card, perhaps you are feeling worn out, bruised by life's circumstances, susceptible to others, or vulnerable to your environment. Take some time to reflect upon any ways that you may give so much energy to others that you deplete your own energy. Observe with whom you do this, noticing your thoughts and feelings and any body awareness. Yarrow has a powerful ability to thrive and to heal. Yarrow may come to you at this time of healing to remind you to avoid overextending your energy on everyone else and to save some energy for yourself. This may be a good time for you to guard all the things that you do and people you serve and just take some time out for yourself. Protect your health, cleanse your thoughts, release your tensions, and detach yourself from the problems of others.

If you are a person who is overexposed to the public daily or who provides healing to others, or if you have job burnout and are feeling overwhelmed, Yarrow is letting you know the importance of protecting your energy and yourself.

Energy Impact *(chakra correspondence)*
7th chakra

Affirmations

"I take personal space to gather my strength and to regain my energy."

"I wrap myself up in my protected cocoon."

"I lovingly detach myself from other people's problems."

"My inner light glows within me and surrounds me."

YELLOW MONKEYFLOWER

(Mimmulus guttatus)

PRIMARY QUALITY: TRUST/OVERCOMING FEAR

Voice of the Flower

"The steady flow of the waters that I live in strengthens my roots as they search deeper for their foothold into the earth below me. I feel a profound fear that my roots will lose hold when the water's force becomes swifter and stronger. I am afraid that its current may sweep me away, yet something inside of me knows that I can relax and go with the water's flow. With trust and confidence, I let go of my fear as I allow the current of the water to move through me and all around me. I allow myself to move with this flow, and as I do, I let go of my fears and sing out my newfound freedom. I give you this opportunity to allow yourself to move forward with the currents of life, letting go of your fears and embracing what is to come."

Insight

When you choose the Yellow Monkeyflower card, you may be on a path of healing that is about overcoming any fears you may have. You may in some way be hiding behind a false mask to cover up your fears and your true expression of self, feeling trapped by life's setbacks and situations. The Yellow Monkeyflower is a gentle kindred spirit, giving you the trust to believe in yourself. Yellow Monkeyflower is here to feed you strength, letting you express your uncertainties without fear in everyday experiences. Allow yourself to flow with the natural currents in life that feed your soul. Take in the confidence and trust Yellow Monkeyflower gives to you, releasing your fears and facing your unbound freedom. Enjoy your journey!

Energy Impact (chakra correspondence)
1st, 2nd, 3rd, and 5th chakras

"Facing my fears with strength and confidence, I embrace my freedom."

"I allow myself to express my feelings and fears with those whom I know I
can trust."

"I allow the water of my body to cleanse away my fears."

YERBA SANTA

(Eriodictyon Angustifolium)
PRIMARY QUALITY: THE SACRED WITHIN

Voice of the Flower

"I invite you to embrace and honor your body as a sacred temple. From within
your temple spaces, I offer you cleansing and purification. In this place, you
are given the opportunity to sort out and discover whatever impurities are
causing you to shut down, preventing you from well-being. As you cleanse
yourself of that which holds you back, you will feel a renewal of energy and
strength filled with Divine love and light-filled radiance. May your renewed
self inspire you to step forth and follow through with your life's choices, honoring your body and your mind, as you live your path of wholeness."

Insight

When you choose the Yerba Santa card, you may in some way be feeling shut
down. Yerba Santa helps you to reach into the depths of your inner world,
sorting out any impurities from within to without, finding your pathway of
healing. By doing so, you will experience more strength in your character,
acceptance, and determination to look within in order to heal your whole
person. Prepare some time to be with yourself, and contemplate on one thing
about yourself that you might call an "impurity," such as something that goes
very deep and probably feels buried. Try to pick it up and look at it very carefully. Feel it, touch it, listen to what it has to say. Ask what you can do for it.

Yerba Santa guides you to follow through with your outer tasks as you meet your inner needs. Perhaps Yerba Santa will inspire you to eat cleansing foods, drink cleansing beverages, give thoughtful prayers, and take good care of yourself. You just might notice how the world around you changes as you do.

Energy Impact (chakra correspondence)
7th chakra (indirectly 5th chakra—physical throat conditions)

Affirmations
"I give thanks to myself and my ability to rediscover my lost parts."

"I pray that I will heal in body, mind, and soul and that all impurities will come out in the open and be seen, heard, and touched."

"I take full responsibility to follow through with life's tasks/(name a particular task for you) and to make an achievable goal of completion."

"I honor the Sacred within myself."

YUCCA (SOAPTREE)

(Yucca elata)
PRIMARY QUALITY: SPEAR OF DESTINY

Voice of the Flower
"I stand with great endurance as my roots burrow deep within the earth below and as my stalk reaches to meet the sky above. I am protected all around my base with spiny-tipped and fibrous leaves which can be used to make cordage and baskets. I am a very useful plant. Many parts of me are cleansing, and the taste of my flowers is divine. You will notice that my creamy-colored flowers rise in clusters toward the top of my stalk and bloom even in the darkest of the night. I offer you my shining light to help you stay focused on your life's dreams and your life purpose. May you gather the strength and endurance needed to move forward in your life, and may your determination

be free of entanglements. Prayerfully ask for Divine guidance and I will shed light upon your journey."

Insight

When you choose the Yucca card, your path of healing may be calling you to take a look at the practical ways you invest your time and how you accomplish everyday tasks. Are these tasks leading you toward your goals in life? Yucca helps you stay focused on your life's work, giving you endurance, strength, and determination with softness and gentleness. Perhaps you will tap into the enormous power of the Yucca, feeling its fullness and feeling empowered to take actions that will help you move forward in life. Let the light of the Yucca shine upon you, giving meaning and hope in your life, and guide you on your journey.

Energy Impact (chakra correspondence)
7th chakra

Affirmations

"May the seeds of my dreams guide my path and destiny."

"I have the strength, endurance, determination, and wisdom to stay focused on my life's path."

"I choose to take actions that will help me to move forward in my life."

BEYOND THE FLORAL CARPET

Silently I sit on soft grasslands
surrounded by Mother Earth's rainbow-colored floral blanket.
I feel the warmth of the sun against my face and
observe the sunlight glistening through the crystal bowl at my feet.

An infusion of Air-Fire-Water-Earth sparks
a creation of Divine Alchemy,
bringing forth a mystery of Nature.

The flowers' fragrance beholds their secrets.
Their enriching colors behold their beauty.
Their unique signatures behold a personality and expression.
The taste of their nectar beholds their essence.
A whole plant journey with a flower beholds a silent presence that heals the
Soul.

Oh subtle essence of the flowers,
my mind in Silence listens to your prayers and voices
and seeks the wisdom that you share.

I am awakened to your secrets
through my senses.

You have touched me, a doorway opens.

GOING DEEPER

In this section we'll look at each of the seven chakras and the specific areas of the body with which they are associated. Each of the seven chakras also corresponds, energetically, to a color. When we work with the chakras we say that each area or energy center in your body is filled with a color of the rainbow, beginning with red, then layered with the colors of orange and yellow, then green at the center, followed by blue, then violet, with white/gold which emanates all around the rainbow's arch.

THE SEVEN CHAKRAS AND THEIR COLORS
A PATHWAY OF WHOLENESS

The First Chakra—Red

The root or first chakra in the human body is located between the base of the spine or tailbone known as the coccyx and the pubic bone. It includes the functions of the anus, rectum, circulatory system, reproductive system which includes the testicles and the ovaries, the gonads (sex glands), the kidneys, and the lower extremities such as the feet, legs, and the entire pelvic area.

The root chakra has a grounding energy, connecting you to the earth and helping you build the foundation of yourself. It is an innate primal energy and the vital root of your spiritual and soul heritage. The root chakra is the foundation of where you have come from and indicates what way you are going to develop. The root chakra is about survival and power. It includes your awareness and needs of the physical world such as food, shelter, clothing, exercise, and nutrition, yet it also includes a deeper unconscious awareness that takes you back to the very roots from which you came.

90

The root chakra is also the seat of the kundalini or life force energy and affects the way you breathe and move. The serpent represents the expression of the kundalini life force energy and is associated with both masculine and feminine traits. A common symbol in the medical field is represented by the two serpents (male and female) which intertwine together along a caduceus or staff. In other systems, the serpents symbolize a mystical awakening of hot and fiery kundalini energy. This energy rises from the base of the spine and aligns with all of your energy centers to the crown chakra at the top of the head. Experiencing the kundalini brings harmony, balance, and an incredible feeling of flowing life force energy.

The color associated with the root chakra is red, the first color in the rainbow spectrum and a color associated with the element of earth.

The Second Chakra—Orange

The second chakra connects with the reproductive system, including the prostate and sex organs, which are responsible for the production of estrogen, progesterone, sperm, and testosterone. It is also connected with the lower back and the body's muscular system. The second chakra includes the partial functions of the adrenal glands, the lymphatic glands, the spleen, bladder, pancreas, and kidneys. This center also affects the process of elimination and detoxification of the body. If you think about what water represents in the body, this makes sense. Drinking plenty of water feeds your organs and your blood, helping you function fluidly.

Water symbolizes your emotions. Emotions are a driving force which gives you the incentive to get where you want to go and to help you get in touch with how you feel about who you are. When you begin to understand the emotions of fear, anger, grief, and guilt, why you feel them, and where they came from, you can then put these feelings into their proper perspective. Your emotions flow like the current in the river depending upon the driving force of energy moving through you. You learn to yield as the tide and to flow as the river, continually releasing, cleansing, changing, and evolving. You are constantly pulled between the release of letting go of old feelings and emotions that limit you, that prevent personal growth, and possibly that blame others for your suffering, and toward the pull of moving in a whole new way that can free you from the bondage of your feelings and stuck patterns while requiring a new identity of yourself.

When you have come to terms with emotional attachments that have held you in bondage, you begin to prepare yourself for a new relationship with yourself. Learning how powerful your emotions are and the energetic impact they have on both yourself and others can help you use them as effective tools, teaching you about who you are and who you want to become.

The second energy center holds the key to your personal investment in yourself, to your creativity and the birth of new emotional patterns and ideas, and to your ability to take care of and nurture yourself and others. By discovering yourself through your emotional world, you can uncover inner treasures of harmony, balance, and peace. And most important, you can begin to feel a new sense of trust, as you come to know who you are. You develop confidence, endurance, and emotional security.

The second energy center is also the center of sexuality and sensation. As you come into a new identity of yourself, you experience a sense of freedom and creativity which can include a newfound relationship with your own sexuality. You begin to learn new steps in the dance of life that stir your passion and excitement for living. You find yourself accepting and embracing life's setbacks, and you begin to evolve into a new style of living that supports who you are and what you have established in the foundation of your being.

The second chakra is associated with the color orange, the second color in the rainbow spectrum, which is also associated with the element of water.

The Third Chakra—Yellow

The third energy center of the human body is located in the solar plexus area. Its functions include the adrenals, stomach, digestive system, assimilation process, liver, and gall bladder. This center is also associated with the left hemisphere of the brain and its activities. Mentally unbalanced or psychosomatic illnesses, ulcers, and intestinal/digestive malfunctions can be relieved by healing work in this center.

The third chakra is the energy center which gives you your ability to reason, to find purpose in life, and to empower yourself to be who you need to be. Awareness of your third energy center can help you to understand your thought dialogues in relation to your feelings. It can strengthen your mind so you develop a state of stability, courage, faith, hope, humor, and joy. This energy center brings about a balanced mental state of responsibility, objectivity, and wisdom. Awareness of this center can help you to surrender the mind when needed. It also links the rational mind to psychic energies and enhanced intuition. It can give you the courage and faith to act upon and trust in your intuition. The third energy center reveals a higher consciousness that is contained within the lower three chakras. This consciousness has an innate capability to understand yourself and others. It is the bond between the lower chakras (your root, emotions, and mind) and the heart, uniting love and harmony, de-crystallizing old patterns.

The third energy center is the place where you come to terms with who you are, what you have come here to learn, and what you truly desire. It is the beginning of your journey with yourself, and as you honor your true self, you will be guided on the path of self-empowerment and dignity.

By working with your thought patterns in this energy center, you can dissolve prejudice, judgment, and criticisms. You can learn how to effectively deal with anger, understand your hatred and where it has rooted, and dissolve and unplug from your rational and irrational fears.

93

A conscious and healthy relationship to the solar plexus chakra helps you to trust your intuition and the guidance you may receive from the higher chakras. This chakra center is complemented by the violet-purple ray of the sixth chakra, which indicates your ability to receive higher aspirations and to allow spiritual guidance and vision to flow through you.

The third chakra is connected with the color yellow, the third color in the spectrum of the rainbow. Yellow is associated with the element of fire, the warmth of the sun, the way that you think, and the power of your mind.

The Fourth Chakra—Pink and Green

The center chakra is the heart center which is the bridge or connector between the three lower energy centers and the three higher energy centers. The heart chakra includes the functions of the heart, the thymus gland, the immune system, and the circulatory system. This center is also associated with the right hemisphere of the brain and with tissue regeneration.

As the marriage of the three upper and the three lower chakras, the heart center is where Communication, Vision, Light, Wisdom, and Higher Consciousness from above meet with Matter, Survival, Procreation, Emotions, Knowledge, and Personality from below. When the upper and lower chakras are balanced and their energy currents are freely flowing, the heart chakra radiates a creative force of energy, power, and unconditional love.

Here, the merging of sexuality with the true expression of sexual love is generated and the passion of mystical awakening is stirred. The heart center is the focal point where your personal development reaches a new stage of growth. This is experienced and demonstrated by your greater ability to allow your heart to dictate which choices you make. Your heart center becomes open to a higher expression of love, compassion, and willpower. As this naturally unfolds, you become more open, experiencing a universal, unconditional love that expands well beyond yourself, your family, and your friends.

It is at the heart center or heart chakra where you offer healing of your own emotional wounds that may date as far back in your history as you can remember or even beyond your conscious memories. It is at this center where you offer healing, forgiveness, and love for self and others. You come to realize that you no longer need to feed negative energies or limiting beliefs about yourself or others, and you learn to bless and love others while staying on your own path.

The colors associated with the heart chakra are pink and green. Pink is the union between the root chakra, associated with the color red, and the seventh energy center at the top of your head, which is associated with the color white. Green is a mixture of yellow (third energy center) and blue (fifth energy center). Green is also the color in the middle of the rainbow, thus its association with the heart, the center in our bodies where we feel love, compassion, and forgiveness.

The Fifth Chakra—Blue

The fifth chakra is located around the throat and is associated with sound, vibration, and communication. The throat energy center includes the throat, larynx, tongue, mouth, lips, teeth, esophagus, thyroid, and the parathyroid glands. It also includes the activities of the respiratory system, bronchial and vocal functions, and the processing and absorption of foods/nutrients. The throat chakra is also associated with the upper extremities—neck, shoulders, arms, and hands.

The throat chakra is where you receive the higher vibratory frequencies of the sixth and seventh chakras and connect those frequencies with the heart. The throat chakra is the energy center of spiritual willpower. As you become more open to embrace the Light and the higher energy currents within yourself, you spontaneously bring spiritual guidance and vision into your cognitive mind—in both thoughts and images. You are better able to bring in positive thought forms and attitudes. An opening or awakening of the throat energy is indicated by your ability to speak your truths from an inner depth of awareness, spiritual guidance, and a place of compassion within your heart. Communication takes place not only through the expression of vocal exchange, but through the expression of creative art forms such as dance, sculpture, painting, singing, sound, chanting, playing instruments, and language.

The expression of communication is the passage of your inner self (your voice, its sounds and vibrations, your thoughts, inner truths and insights) to the outside world and the responses that are returned to you. You become more aware of yourself and even get to know yourself better by observing and listening to the ways you communicate and to the ways others respond to your communication.

The throat chakra is commonly related to the color blue.

The Sixth Chakra—Violet-Purple

This chakra is known as the third eye, ajna, or brow chakra. It is located slightly above and between the eyes, and it is associated with the pineal gland and endocrine system. The brow chakra is also associated with the immune system: the eyes, ears, sinuses, and face; and the synapses of the brain. This energy center helps provide the balance between the left and right hemispheres of the brain.

The third eye or brow chakra is the visionary energy center which gives you wisdom and spiritual insight. On a more personal level, the brow chakra is the energy center that teaches you about judgment, truth, honesty, and integrity and how your mind responds to your truths. This center empowers you to acknowledge and identify your wisdom and to act according to the wisdom you receive. It frees stagnation and helps you to define purpose and spiritual understanding. It also enables you to allow Light to come through your third eye and to receive the message/s that the Light brings. The third eye is the vibrational point where the darkness from the center of the earth and the Light from the center of the sun merge together as one. The light and darkness together create a balanced sixth chakra. This energy center works with the mental aspects of the third chakra and allows a higher consciousness and spiritual vision to direct your mental thought forms.

Your awareness into the third-eye energy center gives you the ability to internally see your memories, dreams, thought forms, and imagination. It is at this center where you take in, hold, clarify, create, and manifest visual information. This chakra opens the gateway in your ability to step beyond yourself and to obtain the higher power that is already inherently within you. It opens you toward clairvoyant and psychic awareness—to the ability to see beyond time and space. Your awareness into this energy center will help you access information and perception from within your mind's eye that gives you details about a person, place, or event. You probably have experienced this center in your life in various ways. An example may include thinking about a person such as your mother, or a friend, right before the phone rings and it is that person. You may see lights, color, images, and even your emotions or the emotions or energy fields of others. It is through this energy center that you gain access to long-distance healing by sending your prayers and healing to others in the absence of their physical presence.

This energy center awakens your intuition and your insights at a deep level. It gives you the power to tap into a higher vibrational frequency that is linked with the collective unconscious. It is through the powerful connection of the collective unconscious that your energy is shared and united.

The sixth chakra is associated with the sixth color of the rainbow spectrum, violet-purple.

The Seventh Chakra—White

The seventh energy center within the human body is known as the crown chakra. The crown chakra is located at the top of the head. It is associated with the cerebral cortex, the central nervous system, the pituitary gland, and all the pathways of the nerves and electrical synapses within the body.

The seventh chakra energy center is associated with both conscious and unconscious thoughts. These thoughts include your belief systems, how you see yourself, how you see others, and how you look at and examine events in your life.

Experiencing the seventh chakra is spontaneous and effortless. The seventh chakra aligns you with your spiritual essence and with an intrinsic knowing that is linked to your higher consciousness. Higher consciousness relates to a broader understanding or relationship with yourself and the Divine Power that is bigger than, yet inclusive of, the physical world and your experiences in it. Consciousness includes your ability to live in the here and now, to plant the seeds of Divine Intelligence in your thoughts, and to nurture these seeds so they will be made manifest. Consciousness comes from a place inside of yourself that allows you to reach for and obtain higher knowledge.

As you gain access to your crown chakra, you will discover a boundless eternity that allows you to be nowhere yet everywhere all at once. The crown chakra energy center is where you explore, study, and experience an expansion of information. You'll be able to view reruns of your belief and value systems, the way you see yourself and your internal patterns, the way you interact in the world at large, the way you receive information, and the way you truly evolve into your spirituality.

By working with the seventh chakra, you become more aware of your relationship with a Divine Power. When you consciously devote time each day to be in the silence of your mind, with the presence of the Sacred, you become one with the purpose of your life's work. On an energetic level, you may begin to experience the connection between your heart and throat energy centers. You may begin to feel a vibrant energy flow throughout your body and all around you. You can become more and more conscious of this system of energy within yourself and discover more about how it works to create who you are. You may find that you begin to see yourself as a vibrant and flowing system of energy, mindful of every situation you find yourself in and of the way you hold or give away power. It is at this place where you feel as One with all of Creation—expanded, connected, and at peace with the Divine Power within yourself and with all life-forms.

The crown chakra is related to white, white light, and the top of the rainbow spectrum, which often has a gold glow surrounding it.

The following chart will be a handy reference for you, showing the correspondence between the chakras, their elements, colors, and flower essences. See page 103 for more about working with flower essences.

As you become more familiar with this subtle energy system, you will begin to experience the chakras centers as a road map. And as you work on your navigating skills, you will get to know how each part of the system works with the others to form a whole. The more you become aware of these energy (power) centers within you, the greater your synthesis will be. You will find yourself more balanced and able to feel, act, think, and be a whole person.

Blessings on your journey.

Chakra	Also known as	Element	Focus	Color
1st Chakra	Physical, Root, or Base Chakra	Earth	Survival, Physical Security	Red
2nd Chakra	Emotional, Spleen, or Regenerative Chakra	Water	Sexuality, Procreation, Emotions	Orange
3rd Chakra	Mental, Personal Power, or Solar Plexus Chakra	Fire	Will, Purpose, Power, Self-Empowerment, Self-Honor	Yellow
4th Chakra	Heart Chakra	Air	Love, Compassion, Forgiveness	Pink/Green
5th Chakra	Throat Chakra	Ether	Communication, Sound, Vibration	Blue
6th Chakra	Third Eye, Ajna, or Brow Chakra	Radium	Seeing, Visualization, Clairvoyance, Light, Intuition, Psychic Perception, Imagination	Violet/Purple
7th Chakra	Crown Chakra	Magentum	"The Thousand-Petaled Lotus," Bliss, Understanding, Oneness with the Infinite, Peace, Expanded Consciousness, Communication with the Divine	White/Gold

Endocrine Gland	Flower Essences
Adrenals	Black-Eyed Susan / Blanketflower / Bouncing Bet / Century Plant / Crimson Monkeyflower / Desert Willow / Echinacea / Indian Paintbrush / Mexican Hat Paloverde / Peace Rose / Pinyon / Pomegranate / Sage / Saguaro Scarlet Penstemon / Strawberry Hedgehog / Yellow Monkeyflower
Gonads	Blanketflower / Calendula / California Poppy / Century Plant / Crimson Monkeyflower / Echinacea / Indian Paintbrush / Mexican Hat / Mullein / Paloverde / Pomegranate / Scarlet Penstemon Yellow Monkeyflower
Pancreas	Aster / Black-Eyed Susan / Blanketflower / Blue Flag Iris / Calendula / Century Plant / Chamomile / Cliff Rose / Columbine / Comfrey / Desert Marigold Desert Willow / Honeysuckle / Mexican Hat / Mullein / Ox-Eye Daisy Palmer's Penstemon / Paloverde / Pomegranate / Purple Robe / Sage Scarlet Penstemon / Strawberry Hedgehog / Sunflower / Wild Rose Yellow Monkeyflower
Thymus	Bells-of-Ireland / Bouncing Bet / Comfrey / Desert Willow / Evening Primrose Indian Paintbrush / Morning Glory / Onion / Palmer's Penstemon / Peace Rose / Pinyon / Sage / Saguaro / Strawberry Hedgehog / Sweet Pea / Thistle Wild Rose / Willow
Thyroid	Blue Flag Iris / Chicory / Comfrey / Crimson Monkeyflower / Desert Larkspur Desert Willow / Palmer's Penstemon / Sage / Scarlet Penstemon Yellow Monkeyflower / Yerba Santa
Pituitary	Aster / Blue Flag Iris / Chicory / Comfrey / Desert Larkspur / Echinacea Indian Paintbrush / Lupine / Morning Glory / Palmer's Penstemon / Pinyon Purple Robe / Thistle / Vervain
Pineal	Aster / Bells-of-Ireland / Black-Eyed Susan / Blue Flag Iris / Bouncing Bet Chamomile / Cliff Rose / Columbine / Comfrey / Desert Willow Evening Primrose / Honeysuckle / Lupine / Morning Glory / Onion Ox-Eye Daisy / Peace Rose / Sage / Saguaro / Thistle / Vervain / Willow Yarrow / Yerba Santa / Yucca

LIVING FLOWER ESSENCES

Flower essences contain a sacred plant energy which can balance human discord, reestablishing the link between body and soul, nature and spirit. These flower essences are plant helpers that teach us to live life at its fullest with greater self-awareness and connect us with our Divine nature.

Each flower or plant has a unique form, smell, color, texture, taste, and a special "sense" or gift that it will share with others. The flower or plant offers a special message or lesson which arouses a feeling and/or thought unique to the flower's own identity and individualization. Often, the characteristics and personalities of flowers offer a lesson or message exactly at a time when you need it most, helping you to be in touch with your innermost nature.

As you use Living Flower Essences, you will soon experience the powerful yet gentle effects they offer you. Treasure the gifts of these special plants and allow your own personal growth to unfold and blossom.

To utilize the plant's unique energy pattern, flowers are picked and placed in a clear glass bowl of purified water at their peak of blossoming. This is called an infusion. The infusion containing the flower's blossoms is set out in direct sunlight, or in some cases, moonlight.

The energy of the sunlight or moonlight extracts the energy of the blossom into the water and creates a life force pattern which reflects the character of that flower or plant.

This simple method of making a flower essence contains the four natural elements (earth, air, fire (sun), and water) as well as the "essence" of the flower. According to Manly Hall in his book *Paracelsus*, this essence was referred to by the Pythagoreans and Paracelsians as the "quintessence" or "fifth essence," an invisible spiritual energy source that is experienced as an expression of the soul. As a whole, the four elements and the "quintessence" produce a powerful, effective means of healing. The energy pattern of the "quintessence" is stored within the flower essence and can be used for physical, emotional, mental, and spiritual healing.

The flower essence and its vibrational influence with the chakra or energy center may assist you with your inner alignment. You may learn to understand yourself better and to make more conscious choices in your life changes toward your path toward wholeness. As you begin this new relationship with yourself, it will help you to feel connected with the One who lives and breathes through you and as you.

If your vital force is depressed, a root chakra flower essence may help to invigorate you. They are stimulating and warming. If you are having some emotional challenges, second chakra flower essences will help you look at the deeper underlying emotion. They may offer a cleansing effect, helping you to feel more joyful and perhaps more at peace with your emotional body.

When the mental activity of a person is either deficient or in excess, a third chakra flower essence may help to either stimulate or soothe, depending on the flower. Flower essences related to the fourth chakra offer a path of healing for the heart, helping you to release judgments, forgiveness, sadness, and grief.

Flower essences associated with the fifth chakra are usually made with blue flowers which enhance the power of imagination and clarity of thought in the way you communicate, inspiring deeper insights into the ways you create and express yourself. Blue flowers have a quietly soothing yet energetic effect.

The violet-lavender-purple flowers prepared as sixth chakra flower essences offer spiritual vision and inner guidance, enhance imagination, creative visualization, perception, intuition, a deepened awareness, and understanding. Flower essences associated with the seventh chakra are made with white- or cream-colored flowers, offering psychic cleansing, protection, release, insight, and an overall lightness.

Flower essences are nonaddictive and are generally very safe. At Living Flower Essences, we prepare them in a formula with a base of brandy or apple cider vinegar, vegetable glycerin, and pure water. These essences are very dilute and are generally recognized as safe for most people. However, if you have any questions or doubts, please check with your health professional before and during use. Those people with alcoholic problems should avoid the brandy base and request an apple cider vinegar base. Also, these products may not be safe for people who are diabetic due to the vegetable glycerin. A diabetic may want to request apple cider vinegar only as a base.

Flower essences are generally safe for babies, children, animals, and the elderly. If you are giving a flower essence to a small child or an animal, observe the effects and continue or discontinue use based upon the response.

EXPECTATIONS OF FLOWER ESSENCES

104

Flower essences can work subtly or dramatically. You may instantly notice a shift in your awareness, or it may take a few hours or days to observe and feel the effects of flower essences and how they orchestrate change in your life. Flower essences are one tool among many that may help you to seek greater understanding of yourself and all your relations. The more you create time and ceremony with the flowers, the more you will notice their effects.

DOSAGE

Take three to four drops under your tongue two to four times per day, according to your needs and level of sensitivity. You may decide to take the flower essence more frequently (such as six to eight times per day) for the first several days. This may help you to heighten your sensitivity to the flower or plant, and then you can gradually reduce the number of times taken per day according to your own needs. Continue to take the essence as long as you wish. Trust your intuition on this.

You can also add flower essences to bathwater, spray bottles, herbal products, the family water crock, or to your animal's water bowl.

FLOWER ESSENCES FOR PETS AND ANIMALS

Selecting essences for animals is similar to choosing essences for people. You can check for the animal's symptoms and look for similar symptoms in the repertory of essences. I have treated many different types of animals with flower essences, especially birds, cats, dogs, and horses. If you take some time to get to know the flowers and their voices, they will guide you on a path of healing for your pet or animal.

Some common flower essences for pets are the following:

Grief and the loss of a loved one, an owner being out of town — Wild Rose, Peace Rose, and Yarrow.

Aggression (ill-tempered bird who bites or plucks feathers, dog who attacks or bites) — Calendula, Chamomile, Crimson Monkeyflower, Century Plant, Saguaro, and Yarrow.

Fear (loud noises such as thunderstorms, blenders, vacuum cleaners, or fear of strangers) — Century Plant, Yellow Monkeyflower, Calendula, Chamomile, Lupine, Saguaro, and Yarrow.

High-strung and restless animals — Calendula, Chamomile, Vervain.

Trauma — Calendula, Century Plant, Chamomile, Lupine, Saguaro, and Yarrow.

Tired and withdrawn — Blanketflower, Chamomile, Echinacea, Sunflower, Yarrow.

In heat — Calendula and Chamomile.

Difficulty sleeping — Calendula, Yellow Monkeyflower, Saguaro, and Yarrow.

In giving flower essences to animals, the signs will be evident when the flower essence is effective. Generally, you will notice in a matter of minutes or a few hours if a flower essence is working. In some cases, you may need to wait for two or three days. In my experience, most animals have a fairly quick response to the therapeutic effect of flower essences, and you will soon know if a particular essence is working or whether you want to try another essence.

If you feel the essence is working, continue to give the animal the essence for a minimum of three days for an acute condition and a minimum of fourteen days for a chronic condition.

If you feel the essence isn't working, then try another essence and observe the results.

BIBLIOGRAPHY

Bach, Edward, M.D., and F.J. Wheeler, M.D. *The Bach Flower Remedies*. New Canaan, CT: Keats Publishing, Inc., 1977.

Brennan, Barbara Ann. *Hands of Light*. New York: Bantam Books, 1988.

Bruyere, Rosalyn L. *Wheels of Light*. New York: Fireside, 1989, 1991, 1994.

Ellis, Pk. *strata: mapping the voice*. North Vancouver, BC: Gallerie Publications, 1994. Contact information: PK Ellis, P.O. Box 212, Cerrillos, NM 87010 or E-mail: *stratadechelly@yahoo.com*.

Epstein, Ron. *Making and Using Flower Essences*. Los Angeles: Ron Epstein, 1986.

Gimbel, Theo, D.C.E. *Healing Through Color*. Essex, England: The C.W. Daniel Company, Ltd., 1980.

Gladstar, Rosemary. *Rosemary Gladstar's Family Herbal*. North Adams, MA: Storey Publishing, 2001. Visit her website at *www.sagemountain.com*.

Gunther, Bernard. *Energy Ecstasy and Your Seven Vital Chakras*. Van Nuys, CA: Newcastle Publishing Company.

Hall, Manly P. *Paracelsus*. Los Angeles: The Philosophical Research Society Inc., 1964.

Heline, Corinne. *Color and Music in The New Age*. Marina del Rey, CA: DeVorss and Company, 1985.

———. *Healing and Regeneration Through Color*. Marina del Rey, CA: DeVorss and Company, 1983.

Judith, Anodea. *Wheels of Life*. St. Paul, MN: Llewellyn Publications, 1988.

Judith, Anodea and Selene Vega. *The Sevenfold Journey*. Freedom, CA: The Crossing Press, 1993.

Leadbeater, C. W. *The Chakras*. Wheaton, IL: The Theosophical Publishing House, 1927, 5th Printing 1987.

Magley, Beverly. *Arizona Wildflowers*. Billings, MT: Falcon Press Publishing Company, 1991.

Meadows, Kenneth. *The Medicine Way*. Edison, NJ: Castle Books, 2002.

Moore, MariJo. *Tree Quotes*. Candler, NC: Renegade Planets Publishing, 1998. Visit her website at *www.powersource.com/gallery/marijo*.

Myss, Caroline, Ph.D. *Energy Anatomy* cassette tapes. Boulder, CO: Sounds True Publishing, 1996.

PallasDowney, Rhonda. *The Complete Book of Flower Essences.* San Rafael, CA: New World Library, 2002.

Sams, Jamie, and David Carson. *Medicine Cards.* Sante Fe, NM: Bear & Company, 1988.

Sun Bear and Wabun. *The Medicine Wheel: Earth Astrology.* New York: Simon & Schuster Inc., 1992

Vida, Veronica. Unpublished poem. Veronica lives in Clarkdale, Arizona. Veronica has an M.A. in counseling psychology and is an astrologist specializing in children, women, and couples. To schedule a reading, call (928) 634-7302.

Wood, Matthew. *The Book of Herbal Wisdom: Using Plants as Medicine.* Berkeley, CA: North Atlantic Books, 1997.

RESOURCE SECTION

Unless otherwise noted, all of the following products, trainings, and services are available from my company, Living Flower Essences,
P.O. Box 1492, Cottonwood, AZ 86326; (928) 639-3614
Web site: www.livingfloweressences.com
E-mail: info@livingfloweressences.com

The Complete Book of Flower Essences by Rhonda PallasDowney. This book explores the relationships between herbalism, homeopathy, chakras, flower essences, and healing. It can be purchased at *www.amazon.com* or ordered from any bookstore.

Living Flower Essences: The forty-eight flower essences associated with the flower cards featured in this book are available from Living Flower Essences in half-ounce cobalt glass bottles. Our flower essences can be purchased singly, as formulas, or in a Practitioner's Kit that contains all forty-eight flower essences.

Chakra Healing Kit: This kit contains seven flower essences that correspond to the seven chakras, packaged colorfully and including directions. The flower essences in this kit are Indian Paintbrush, Pomegranate, Sunflower, Wild Rose, Desert Larkpsur, Aster, and Saguaro.

Living Flower Essences' Flower Essence and Chakra Healing Practitioner Course: This comprehensive 200 hour certification flower essence course is uniquely designed to offer the student an integration of home study correspondence and a hands on experiential program located in the Verde Valley of Arizona. Call and ask us about other plant healing courses offered.

Nature Retreats and Shamanic Journeys with Curtis and/or Rhonda PallasDowney: Access your inner Power, Wisdom, Abundance, and much more through the development of primitive skills, exploring plant wisdom, and communing with nature. Through mindfulness, nature walks, and ceremony, participants are guided into a greater awareness of their relationships and responsibilities to Self, humanity, and the nature kingdoms.

Women with Wings: Healing Retreats for Women; Co-facilitated by Rhonda PallasDowney and Veronica Vida. Join us in a special retreat located in the serene, rustic setting of a private and exclusive hot springs near Safford, Arizona. Retreat activities and free time are offered to nurture the body and soul.

Living Essence Bottled Water: Flower Essence Infused Water: This special water is made with a flower cocktail of five flower essences: Blanketflower, Aster, Desert Willow, Sage, and Ox-Eye Daisy. For greater enjoyment of this product, you are encouraged to use the affirmations of the flowers. As you drink this water, allow joy, illumination, abundance, integration, and wisdom into your life!

I am also available for private consultations both in person and by phone. Please call (928) 639-3614 to schedule an appointment.

TO OUR READERS

Weiser Books, an imprint of Red Wheel/Weiser, publishes books across the entire spectrum of occult and esoteric subjects. Our mission is to publish quality books that will make a difference in people's lives without advocating any one particular path or field of study. We value the integrity, originality, and depth of knowledge of our authors.

Our readers are our most important resource, and we appreciate your input, suggestions, and ideas about what you would like to see published. Please feel free to contact us, to request our latest book catalog, or to be added to our mailing list.

Red Wheel/Weiser, LLC
P.O. Box 612
York Beach, ME 03910-0612
www.redwheelweiser.com